Living with
tinnitus

DAVID W. REES
and SIMON D. SMITH

Manchester University Press

Manchester and New York

Distributed exclusively in the USA and Canada
by St. Martin's Press

Copyright © David W. Rees and Simon D. Smith 1991

Published by Manchester University Press
Oxford Road, Manchester M13 9PL, UK
and Room 400, 175 Fifth Avenue,
New York, NY 10010, USA

Distributed exclusively in the USA and Canada
by St. Martin's Press, Inc.,
175 Fifth Avenue, New York, NY 10010, USA

A catalogue record for this book is available from the British Library

Library of Congress cataloging in publication data
Rees, David W., 1949-
   Living with tinnitus / David W. Rees and Simon D. Smith.
      p. cm – (Living with)
  Includes bibliographical references.
  ISBN 0-7190-3366-7
  1. Tinnitus—Popular works. I. Smith, Simon D., 1959–
  II. Title. III Series.
  RF293.8.R44 1991
  362.1'978–dc20   91-29743

ISBN
ISBN 0719033667

Typeset in New Century Schoolbook
by Koinonia, Manchester
Printed in Great Britain
by Bell & Bain Ltd, Glasgow

Contents

Preface

This book is written with the intention of helping people suffering from tinnitus and their families.

We know from our work with tinnitus sufferers how the problem can change a happy and outgoing person into a sad and shy individual who feels that no one can help them or even understand their problems. The lack of any outward sign that the person has a problem seems to be just one more frustration. People without tinnitus usually have little awareness or understanding of how disabling a problem it can be and they can seem to be insensitive or even rude. It isn't surprising that many sufferers avoid social situations when so many other people don't seem to care about their problems.

We don't claim to have found a cure for the problem or a method of making those who should know better be more polite and understanding. The approach to tackling tinnitus which we recommend is to show that you can begin to control the problem and ensure that others begin to take account of the additional difficulty that tinnitus brings to life. In short, we want to help you to improve the quality of your life and help those around you to better understand your problem.

The book includes some medical and technical terms with which you may be unfamiliar. We have included a glossary section in the back of the book which explains these terms. We have also included a short section which describes the structure of the ear, which will aid your understanding.

The introductory chapter presents factual information about the condition, its causes, prevalence and treatment, and discusses sufferers' common initial reactions to developing it. There are countless myths and misunderstandings about tinnitus and one of our aims is to help you develop increased knowledge and understanding of this condition.

The second chapter allows the reader to understand and assess the psychological consequences of having tinnitus. It helps the individual reader assess how much interference tinnitus is having in their enjoyment of life. Although all individuals with tinnitus have much in common, we recognise that each individual has a unique experience of tinnitus and its effects. We help each reader assess their unique problem, and on the basis of this assessment point them towards other chapters in the book which will provide strategies for improvements. For us to be successful in helping you overcome the many problems caused by having tinnitus, it is essential that you tackle this and all following chapters in an active way. In a sense, we want to help you become the expert therapist to deal with your unique problem.

Chapters 3, 4 and 5 present self-help treatment approaches to overcoming three of the most common problems caused by severe tinnitus: anxiety, depression and insomnia. The chapters provide well-tried effective strategies that you can tailor to your personal needs. Later in the book there are relaxation techniques which you can practise and benefit from, whether or not you have troublesome anxiety.

Chapter 6 looks at how you change both your internal and external environments to your benefit. It helps you become much more aware of how you can deal effectively with difficult situations. It also looks in some detail at the use of auditory maskers and other external sound sources to block out tinnitus noises.

Chapter 7 provides something that for most sufferers is an innovative approach to overcoming tinnitus. It looks at how your perception of tinnitus noises can be modified and improved by the use of positive imagery to eliminate distress.

We have written the book to demonstrate to the person afflicted by tinnitus that they can resume leading a happy and fulfilled life. We don't want you to simply make the best of it or put up with it, we want you to take active steps to overcome it. We know you can!

David W. Rees
Simon D. Smith

1 Introduction

Chapter goals

By the end of this chapter we hope that you will be able to:

1 Know more than you do now about what tinnitus is, including knowing more about the extent of the problem in terms of how common it is and its various causes.
2 Be familiar with the various treatment approaches available.
3 Recognise and accept the initial emotional reaction you had when your tinnitus first began.
4 Be ready to do something positive about overcoming this problem!

Tinnitus is a medical term for noises in the head or ears that do not originate from outside the body. Whilst it is a common symptom of various ear disorders, it can also occur in the absence of hearing problems and can affect people with no hearing whatever.

The sounds heard

The noises are similar to familiar external sounds but cannot be escaped from as they are from within one's head. Most readers of this book will be all too familiar with the types of tinnitus sounds, but for non-sufferers the British Tinnitus Association have produced an audiotape of very realistic simulated tinnitus sounds. Many non-sufferers to whom we have played the tape, at various volumes, are surprised that tinnitus sufferers are able to lead anything like normal lives. By hearing the tape non-sufferers are able to better appreciate the often awful affliction suffered by some people.

Although the word 'tinnitus' refers literally to the ringing, tinkling or jingling sounds which some sufferers hear, others report differing sounds which range from sounds of running water, often like the waves of the sea, clicking and hissing noises, high pitched whistling noises, often described as like the sound a television set makes when the transmission has just ceased, humming sounds or sounds of a heart beating. About 25% of sufferers hear a pure tone. Some sufferers will hear one sound whilst others may have several.

When the tinnitus sound is heard in precise rhythm with the sufferer's heart beat or pulse it is termed 'pulsatile tinnitus' and may be caused by hearing the flow of blood through larger blood vessels into the head, or may be blood pulsing noisily through the tiny vessels of the inner ear. It does not indicate a serious condition. Approximately one in five tinnitus sufferers have this variety of tinnitus, for which the most effective treatment seems to be auditory masking.

Tinnitus is usually described as being much worse at night, probably because the external sounds more commonly heard during the day effectively mask the tinnitus sounds to some extent.

How common a problem is it?

A number of surveys have been undertaken both in the U.K. and elsewhere to determine how common a problem tinnitus is. Surveys in this country seem to agree that approximately one in five or one in six people experience or have experienced tinnitus sounds which last more than five minutes. Most are not troubled by the sounds (usually because they are either very infrequent or have spontaneously permanently disappeared). The Medical Research Council survey in 1981 of tinnitus symptoms within four major cities found that 2% of people asked complained of 'severe annoyance' and approximately 1 in every 200 said that tinnitus stopped them from leading a normal life. Five per cent of the adult population surveyed reported that tinnitus caused sleep disturbance. American surveys have reported even higher levels of both prevalence and distress but these differences may be due to the different questions and criteria used in the surveys.

The condition is much more common in older people, the peak incidence occurring in those aged over 50. For unknown reasons it is more common in females, which is not explained away by there being more elderly females than males. About half of sufferers have tinnitus in one ear only (more frequently the left ear) and half report the sounds as being in both ears or present somewhere in the middle of their head.

It has been estimated that 300,000 people in the UK suffer from tinnitus to the extent that it severely interferes with their daily lives. However, despite its extent both in terms of degree of suffering and numbers of sufferers, it has failed to enter into most people's awareness. Much of the neglect may be attributed to it being a 'silent' condition, a rather unfortunate description perhaps, but one which reflects its very private nature. There are no external signs of illness and for most sufferers the distress caused may be considered psychological because of its adverse effects on thinking, mood and behaviour.

Causes

Tinnitus arises from a number of causes, some of which are known and understood. Some individuals may have tinnitus for which no cause is apparent. It is important to have each individual's tinnitus investigated because some forms may be treated very effectively, with a minority actually permanently cured. Another important reason is that deterioration in tinnitus (and often the accompanying hearing problem) may be prevented by identifying the cause.

The most common causes are wax in the outer ear, or thickening of the bones around the window, middle and inner ear (otosclerosis). Tinnitus may be caused by frequent exposure to extreme noise. Many people who fortunately do not go on to develop tinnitus will experience noises in their ears after exposure to loud noise from sources such as gunfire, pneumatic drills and so on. The noises often last for only a few seconds or minutes at most. However, it is wise to avoid frequent exposure to loud noise, by the use of protective devices.

Tinnitus may also be brought on by the use of certain medications. A number of commonly used drugs act on the inner ear causing temporary or permanent tinnitus and hearing loss. Meniere's disease has also been cited as a cause of this condition through its physical distortion of the hearing mechanism.

Clearly no one stated cause for tinnitus is all-embracing and for some individuals several causes may be found, whilst for others the origin of their condition will remain a mystery.

Treatment of tinnitus

Tinnitus is a symptom of many different disorders with various causes. The first step in any treatment regime is to attempt to determine the cause of the condition. Some causes can be treated with resultant eradication or reduction of the tinnitus.

Unfortunately, for the majority of tinnitus sufferers there is no effective cure. Advances have been made in recent years in the use of tinnitus maskers and this has become one of the most popular and successful treatment approaches to date.

Tinnitus maskers are devices which are built to produce a band of noise of sufficient frequency content and intensity to mask or cover up the tinnitus sounds. The kind of noise generated by the masker is matched to the intended wearer's requirements and in many cases effective tinnitus control will be obtained. However, it is important to return to the issuing clinic at regular intervals to have progress (or lack of it) monitored, particularly as it is common for those issued with such devices to stop using them if relief is not achieved quickly. Some patients report that they are most effective when used at night on retiring to bed as this is a time when their home is most silent and their tinnitus sounds most troublesome. Maskers are usually worn within or behind the ear, although some models are designed for bedside use to aid sleep. Tinnitus masker use and benefits are described more fully in Chapter 6.

Drugs have not proved, to date, to be terribly useful in alleviating the problem as often their side effects outweigh possible benefits. AM 101 INJECTION

Sufferers have turned to other forms of help such as acupuncture (for which there is no substantial evidence of benefit), biofeedback techniques which assist by helping the sufferer to relax, and homeopathic preparations which seem most effective in helping the relaxation process and are preferable to having to take tranquillisers. Changes in diet seem to have no direct effect on tinnitus. Others have turned to hypnotherapy which can be beneficial in helping sufferers come to terms with tinnitus.

Experiments began almost two hundred years ago on the possible therapeutic value of electrically stimulating the ear. For some time we have witnessed the benefits patients with severe pain can derive from the use of electrical stimulators which can effectively block pain sensations.

It is still very early days yet in the application of these approaches for people with tinnitus and much has to be learned about safe use and the optimum sites for electrode placement. Doctors have found that stimulation of the cochlea with very weak electrical currents for short periods of time can be helpful, although to date the effects are short-lived. It is possible that this approach might be of use to those with tinnitus who are profoundly deaf and who therefore cannot benefit from the use of auditory maskers.

Initial reactions to developing tinnitus

Sometimes patients who have tinnitus feel angry, upset or confused about the problem. They sometimes repeat the same questions 'why me?' or 'will I ever get over it?' Sometimes it helps them to think about their problem in a way that is a bit more familiar to them.

The sad fact is that most of us have lost someone close to us. Although it may not seem to be similar at first, mourning the loss of someone close to us is much the same as coming to terms with tinnitus. This is because grief can follow any loss if the thing which has gone holds great personal or emotional importance. This can mean not only the death of a person but also of a much loved pet, or even the theft of an object with great sentimental value. The loss of a limb can cause grief, so the possible loss of something as important as good hearing will also have an emotional cost.

Why is it helpful to think of grief in relation to tinnitus distress? Firstly, it helps the sufferer to recognise and accept their emotions, and second, it helps them to have hope for the future. It is a painful and unpleasant process, but it is also a process that can be worked through successfully. In addition, it can be recognised as a natural process which has an end point. The end of the process is not that the loss is made good, but that the person is able to accept their changed state. They are also more easily able to accept that others have been through a similar sadness and are now able to find pleasure in their lives, although they may admit that they still notice their loss and it continues to occasionally upset them.

The process of coming to terms with loss can be thought of as a journey which begins with the person accepting that they have a problem and ends with them being able to accept the problem as being a part of their lives. It is important to recognise that this does not mean that the person likes the new situation, only that they can have a successful life in spite of it. The problem with being angry about having tinnitus is that constant rage about the unfairness of something which cannot be changed can become destructive to the person and those around them and can then destroy relationships.

Anger is like an acid, it starts to eat away at the person who made it, then spreads to those closest. The best way to use it is to remove the cause. Start to solve the problems, not give yourself more. Remember, it's often easier to stay angry than to find out why.

Tasks

1 Accept that the problem has happened to you.
2 Cope with the upset that this will cause.
3 Adjust to the change that has happened.
4 Begin to plan for a future that will include your problem, but will still be well worth enjoying.

Learn to live with it!

Most sufferers will be told by their doctors that they must learn to live with it. The central purpose for writing this this book is to help you do just that. Whilst all sufferers may hope and pray that their tinnitus will one day spontaneously disappear (and for some it will), the chances are that it will remain as a potent means of reducing the quality of your life. The central aim is to ensure that you lead the best possible quality of life you can, however interfering in your life tinnitus has been to date. We are not advocating that you simply put up with it. We do not recommend passive acceptance. We want to help you take active steps to overcome it.

2 Assessment for action

Chapter goals

This chapter is a key section of the book. It is a long chapter with many ideas and concepts which might be new to you. It will take quite a while to read and the assessment of the problems you have because of tinnitus needs to be done with care and thought. Take your time to work through the chapter. By the end of the chapter we hope that you will:

1 Be even more willing than you are now to tackle the problems associated with your tinnitus.
2 Recognise that success lies in your hands; you will be the one that determines how successful you are.
3 Recognise how preoccupied you may have become with your experience of tinnitus.
4 Be able to assess whether your tinnitus is disrupting your sleep, or causing you anxiety or depression.
5 Recognise that your experience of tinnitus varies from time to time and that you can understand why this should be so.

This chapter has been written to help you, in many ways, become your own therapist. We recognise that whilst all tinnitus sufferers have much in common, they also are individuals with their own specific and personal set of problems. We have written this book to ensure that you can examine the problems caused by your experience of tinnitus, and find within the book tried and tested effective strategies to overcome the problems it causes you.

Many readers of this book will have had tinnitus for many years and will have tried various forms of help, occasionally with some temporary benefit. Many of you will be on the point of giving up all hope of finding relief. Our first goal is to ensure that you do not give up hope and are willing to try again to overcome your tinnitus.

We shall start by looking at your motivation to 'have a go' at tackling your tinnitus problem. We have drawn up a 'framework

Table 2.1 A framework for action: should I try?

Option	Payoffs	Costs
Do nothing (or make a half-hearted effort)	It won't take any effort	I haven't given myself a chance to improve
	I won't be upset by failure	People will blame me for not trying
	Keep my excuse for avoiding situations I I wish to avoid	My tinnitus will remain
Try to follow the advice given in the book	Will have hope that things will improve	Will require a great deal of effort
	Will gain some personal feeling of control over tinnitus rather than vice versa	May not be as successful as I hope
	Improved sense of well-being and self-confidence	Will require time to study and practise new ways
	Able to be and feel normal and not an outsider	Will have disappointments
	Will feel that I have tried to take every opportunity to improve	
	Gain a substantially better quality of life	

for action' which addresses two options.

The two options are that you 'do nothing' (or worse still make a half-hearted attempt to tackle your problem) or 'try to follow the advice given in the book'. Next in the framework for action are two columns: 'payoffs' and 'costs'. These may be thought of as 'positive' and 'negative' or 'plus' and 'minus' consequences of choosing a particular option.

Whenever you are given choices or options it is expected that you will make a decision. Rational decision making is usually based on a comparison between the payoffs and costs of one option and the payoffs and costs of an alternative option. Initially the framework for action (or decision matrix) is blank. In Table 2.1 we have completed the chart with answers given by some of our own patients with tinnitus.

The completed framework is taken from examples provided by our own patients. Whilst some of the items may be true for you too, it is important that you consider what your responses would be. We have provided an empty framework (Table 2.2) for you to complete. It is well worth your taking some time over thinking about this and you may find it helpful to ask other people who know you well for help in completing it.

Table 2.2 My personal framework for action: should I try?

Option	Payoffs	Costs
Do nothing (or make a half-hearted effort)		
Try to follow the advice given in the book		

The next step in the process of using the framework for action is to decide whether items in the payoffs and costs columns are all of equal importance or whether some are more important. In choosing between the two options here, you must take these 'weightings' into account. For example, if you have decided that the 'I haven't given myself a chance to improve' item in the 'costs of doing nothing' column is very important then you will be unlikely to decide to 'do nothing'. Similarly, if you decide that 'being able to feel normal and not an outsider' is of critical importance then you may well choose to 'follow the advice given in the book'.

Once you have chosen (hopefully) to have a go at following advice in this book then we need to see whether the costs of choosing this option can be eliminated or reduced in importance. For example, by choosing to have a go you anticipate (by your responses in the 'costs' column) having to make a great deal of effort and will experience some disappointments. How will you overcome these? Perhaps you should remind yourself that if any improvement occurs it will be worth all the effort and that some of the benefit in following the advice is that the achievements will be of your own making and hence more valuable. You may perhaps console yourself by accepting that there will be disappointments but that these will be far outweighed by the benefits, particularly by the prospect of gaining a substantially better quality of life.

Have a look at the 'costs' for trying to follow the advice in the book that you have listed. Try to work out ways of reducing, or better still eliminating, these few costs. For example, you may well have some disappointments but perhaps you can be consoled by reminding yourself of the achievements attained and the successes to come if you continue 'making an effort'. At worst you might consider that they are a small price to pay for success.

The next step is to consider the 'payoffs' you anticipated by not trying. By trying to follow the advice you are denying yourself these payoffs. How will you deal with these potential losses? One payoff identified by our patients is of having a ready-made excuse to avoid situations. If you try to follow the advice given in the book you may well discover that the number and range of situations that you have in the past wished to avoid becomes considerably reduced. Yes, there will be situations you wish to avoid. This is true of all of us. Maybe part of the action programme that you should consider following is to learn to be honest and assertive and say "thank you for asking me but I do not want to come". Have a look at the payoffs you identified for 'doing nothing'; can they be reduced or eliminated?

An additional step may be to consider your answers to the following two questions, bearing in mind that most readers will not be troubled by tinnitus sounds all of the time.

Question 1 Describe your life when tinnitus is present and troublesome.

Question 2 Describe your life when you are free of tinnitus or when it is less troublesome.

We have asked these two key questions to many of our patients. Whatever the actual content of the two answers, the most striking feature is always the sharp contrast between the two.

Anne described her life with tinnitus as a living hell from which she could find no escape except when asleep, and falling to sleep was difficult without the use of sleeping pills. She described the periods when she was free of tinnitus (very infrequently for her) as bliss and almost like heaven. When free of tinnitus she was carefree, confident and relaxed but for most of the time she was tormented by her tinnitus sounds which she described as like an electric drill boring through her brain. She was low in mood and extremely anxious. Her self-confidence disappeared and she described her life as not worth living.

Some of our patients find it difficult to imagine long periods free of tinnitus but often talk about how wonderful it must be to feel normal, to do the everyday normal things without being under a black cloud.

Write your answers to the two questions in the space provided.

Question 1 Describe your life when tinnitus is present and troublesome.

Question 2 Describe your life when you are free of tinnitus or when it is less troublesome.

Write a list of the benefits or gains you anticipate when you become less handicapped by your tinnitus.

1
2
3
4
5
6
7
8
9
10

It will be useful, from time to time, to remind yourself of your answer to these two questions and to look again at your list (and maybe add to it). In addition, it should prove useful to check back on your framework for action responses in Table 2.2 as you may wish to add new items that have come to mind. You may have realised some additional costs of 'having a go' and it is important to consider how you can steer your way around these rather than be defeated by them.

Unwanted consequences of having tinnitus

The following sections address the unwanted consequences of having tinnitus.

1 Assessment of preoccupation with tinnitus. The first part is an assessment of whether you are particularly preoccupied with having this condition. It consists of two straight forward questions which we would like you to answer as honestly as you can. In addition, we would like you to ask your partner, good friend or close relative to answer the same questions.

Of self
Consider the past month only
1 How much time each day, on average, do you spend talking about tinnitus?
.... minutes each day.

2 How many times in the last seven days have you been preoccupied by your tinnitus?
.... times in the last seven days.

By partner, friend or relative
Consider the past month only
1 How much time each day, on average, does he/she spend talking about his/her tinnitus?
.... minutes each day.

2 How many times in the last seven days has he/she seemed to be preoccupied by his/her tinnitus?
.... times in the last seven days.

The answers to these questions, by yourself and another person, can form part of the basis for assessing the severity of your tinnitus before embarking on the programme outlined in the book. As you improve, we expect that you will become less and less preoccupied with talking about your tinnitus (and spending more and more time enjoying yourself).

2 Assessment of sleep disturbance (insomnia). The majority of our patients complain that tinnitus interrupts their sleep. As mentioned in Chapter 1, 5% of the adult population have had their sleep disturbed at some time by tinnitus. For tinnitus sufferers the proportion with sleep disturbance is probably nearly 100%.

Mary complained of tinnitus sounds which had been present for 15 years. She worked as a clerk in a noisy open-plan office and found that this background noise effectively masked her tinnitus which only became really troublesome when she went to bed at night. She said that as soon as her head hit the pillow it seemed like someone had turned on a steam whistle.

As part of the assessment to examine the adverse effects of tinnitus on your sleep, please complete the following checklist.

Sleep distress assessment
Please circle the number that applies to you for each item
Consider how you have been for the past month only.

1 My tinnitus disturbs my sleep

0	1	2	3	4
Never	Rarely	Sometimes	Most of the time	Always

2 My tinnitus disturbs my sleep by keeping me awake

0	1	2	3	4
Never	Rarely	Sometimes	Most of the time	Always

3 My tinnitus disturbs my sleep by waking me up during the night

0	1	2	3	4
Never	Rarely	Sometimes	Most of the time	Always

4 My tinnitus disturbs my sleep by waking me early in the morning

0	1	2	3	4
Never	Rarely	Sometimes	Most of the time	Always

5 My tinnitus disturbs my sleep so I feel tired in the morning

0	1	2	3	4
Never	Rarely	Sometimes	Most of the time	Always

Add up all your five responses

My total sleep disturbance score is _____

There is no cut-off score between those with problems and those without. Your score measures the extent of the problem with, as you can see, the higher the score the greater the sleep disturbance because of tinnitus. (If it is any comfort, the higher the score, the greater the scope for improvement!)

For sufferers who share a bed or bedroom, their tinnitus (or more correctly, their disturbed sleep) will almost certainly have some unwanted effects on their partner.

Ask your partner to complete the following checklist. It is important that they are honest about how they feel because it is difficult to solve problems if you are unaware of their existence.

The main reason, however, for this exercise is to enlist their support and encouragement. If your problem affects them then so will any improvement you can bring about.

Sleep distress assessment – partner
Please circle the number that applies to you
Consider the past month only.

1 My partner disturbs my sleep

0	1	2	3	4
Never	Rarely	Sometimes	Most of the time	Always

2 My partner disturbs my sleep by keeping me awake

0	1	2	3	4
Never	Rarely	Sometimes	Most of the time	Always

3 My partner disturbs my sleep by waking me up during the night

0	1	2	3	4
Never	Rarely	Sometimes	Most of the time	Always

4 My partner disturbs my sleep by waking me too early in the morning

0	1	2	3	4
Never	Rarely	Sometimes	Most of the time	Always

5 My partner disturbs my sleep so I feel tired in the morning

0	1	2	3	4
Never	Rarely	Sometimes	Most of the time	Always

Add up all your partner's five responses

My partner's total sleep disturbance score is _____

Again, the higher the score the greater the perceived problem. If you decide on the basis of your and/or your partner's score/s that you have a problem worthy of attention, turn to Chapter 5 'Overcoming insomnia' for assistance. The chapter presents well tried and tested means for improving sleep and shows you how to monitor your progress. After a few weeks of making the changes suggested in Chapter 5 it will be worthwhile for you and your partner to complete the two checklists again and compare your scores with your initial ones to demonstrate the progress you will have made.

3 Assessment of anxiety. One of the normal reactions of most people when they are faced with a problem or threat is to become anxious. As you can guess, we find that almost without exception our patients say that they became worried or anxious when they first found that they had tinnitus.

This isn't surprising because an irritating noise suddenly appearing is a frightening experience. The noises trigger off worries about what might be causing it. Although some people seem to adapt to this new situation fairly readily, the majority of people don't seem to become less anxious as time goes on. This may be because although they seek medical treatment a cure cannot be readily found. It is also possible that people don't find the reassurance that they need. They may not be able to find out the cause of their problem. They may not be able to discover whether it will go or possibly become worse. Although it is certainly reassuring to find that the tinnitus doesn't mean that you have a serious physical illness it often isn't enough to stop the worry and anxiety.

When **Geraldine** first heard noises inside her head she thought that she must have something very seriously wrong with her. She thought she could hear blood rushing inside her head. She became more and more upset by this and the noise seemed to get louder. She went to see her family doctor expecting him to confirm that perhaps she had a brain tumour, but he told her that she had developed a condition called tinnitus.

Anxiety, then, becomes a significant problem for the majority of tinnitus sufferers. Anxiety is a word that is used many times a day. People say they are 'anxious' about exams or going for a job interview; they have difficulty sleeping; they have a poor appetite and feel as though they need to use the toilet more than usual.

Although these are all examples of anxiety, it is not really the variety we find amongst our patients. The major difference is that tinnitus sufferers have a constant worry which has been present for weeks, months, or even years!

They feel worn down and often physically exhausted.

They haven't been able to conquer their anxiety which, if anything, seems to be getting worse.

They can't see any hope of improvement.

In addition, they may feel vulnerable or uncomfortable when in company because they have to admit that they can't hear as well as they used to. They sometimes fear that they will become the butt of unkind remarks or may be thought of as stupid.

The examples used previously had a common theme which can go some way towards explaining why even quite severe symptoms can be accepted by the sufferer. The problems are well known, so others would accept that the person had a reason for getting anxious, and try to help. In addition, the person could take comfort from the fact that the problem would be over. He/she may not pass the exam or get the job but at least they could stop worrying about it!

We have included a short questionnaire to assess whether

your tinnitus is causing you undue anxiety. As with the sleep checklist encountered earlier in this chapter, try to answer the questions as honestly as you can by identifying the number which best represents your feelings.

Anxiety assessment

This questionnaire is intended to give you a guide of how anxious you have become.

Fill in the questionnaire by reading the sentences and then putting a circle around the number which best corresponds with how you feel. We realise that the sentences may not be exactly right for you, but please answer each question.

Consider the past month only.

1 I have felt much more on edge than before

0	1	2	3	4
Not at all like me		A little like me		Exactly like me

2 I have been much more short tempered and irritable

0	1	2	3	4
Not at all like me		A little like me		Exactly like me

3 I have begun to worry a lot more about things than I used to

0	1	2	3	4
Not at all like me		A little like me		Exactly like me

4 I haven't been able to relax as easily as I used to

0	1	2	3	4
Not at all like me		A little like me		Exactly like me

5 I haven't felt as confident as I used to be

0	1	2	3	4
Not at all like me		A little like me		Exactly like me

6 I have been waking up several times during the night

0	1	2	3	4
Not at all		A little		Exactly
like me		like me		like me

7 I have found it difficult to go to sleep because my mind has been occupied with problems

0	1	2	3	4
Not at all		A little		Exactly
like me		like me		like me

8 I have been more worried about my general health (not just hearing or tinnitus) than I used to be

0	1	2	3	4
Not at all		A little		Exactly
like me		like me		like me

Add your scores for the eight items

My total anxiety score is _____

Again, the higher the score the higher the level of anxiety and worry induced by having developed tinnitus. Your 'score' can be used for comparison with your score on the same questionnaire after you have spent some time trying out the techniques described and recommended in the book.

The person with tinnitus doesn't often believe that they are going to improve or that any one can help them. They sometimes believe that their problem must have the effect of making their lives terrible.

This doesn't have to be the case. However, it is often quite a struggle before sufferers begin to accept that others have had problems similar to theirs and yet have been able to maintain the quality of the life they used to enjoy.

We can strongly recommend some techniques to help you become more relaxed. The relaxation techniques we endorse are described at the end of the book (pp. 98-105). The exercises are based on progressive muscle relaxation and have been widely practised successfully to eradicate tension. The version on pp. 103-5 is an abbreviated version of that described on pp. 98-105. You should try both and find out which is more suitable for you. It should be said that relaxation exercises are not only of benefit for those with tension but are pleasurable for all of us.

Anxious people are seen by others to be tense and on edge; therefore, learning to relax your muscles makes you seem to be less tense. It has other advantages. Not only do you learn to notice when you are starting to become tense (because you know the difference between tense and relaxed muscles) but you have a skill which will help you to combat the tension.

Whilst straightforward relaxation techniques are invaluable, they are rarely sufficient in themselves. In Chapter 3, 'Overcoming anxiety', we describe a range of techniques and strategies that are 'user-friendly' and have been found, by our patients, to offer solutions to what they have often regarded as insurmountable problems.

4 Assessment of depression. Many of our patients say that they haven't felt the same since their tinnitus became a problem. When we ask them to explain, they say that they feel 'low' or that they can't seem to get as much pleasure from life as they did. They often say that they have given up activities (or are seriously thinking of doing so), not because they are physically unable to continue but because they feel too unhappy or don't see the point of keeping up their interest. Many of them say that they are 'depressed' and their husband or wife agrees that they have changed as a result of their hearing problems.

Depression seems to be an everyday word, we have all used it about ourselves or someone else at one time or another. The problem is that unlike many medical words that people complain that they don't understand, 'depression' is one that everyone seems to understand. Indeed, it is so well known that most people don't realise that it is a medical diagnosis. Of course, when used in the 'everyday' way it doesn't mean that the person is suffering from a mental illness. The problem is that if a person is already feeling 'a bit low', telling themselves (or being told by someone who is trying to help) that they are depressed only adds to the problem.

Depressed people, like anxious individuals, can be often noticed by others as being anxious or depressed. The depressed person may complain that they are depressed, or may give an indication of low mood. However, as we have said, the way that a depressed person acts, the things that they do, make other people who know them well ask them how they are feeling or ask others how they can help.

What do depressed people do which tells others that they may be suffering from low mood?

Try to think of some of the things that you would notice:

1

2

3

4

5

6

We have drawn up a short questionnaire or checklist, later in this section, to assess how depressed you are. The items included are based upon our patients' experiences of depression and include some of the commoner symptoms they report. The symptoms presented in the checklist is not intended to be a complete list of possible effects of depression.

How did you do? Were you able to think of six answers?

Did you think of someone that you know who has been depressed?

Did you try to imagine what you would do if your mood was low?

Did you just write down some of the things that you are feeling at the moment?

If you just wrote down some of the things that you are feeling, you did so because you feel yourself to be in low mood or actually depressed. However, as we said above, people use the word 'depressed' to describe many types of problems. Therefore, we have included a checklist which you can complete to see if your mood is depressed.

Depression assessment

This questionnaire is intended to give you a guide of the degree to which you may have become low in yourself or unduly pessimistic about the future.

Fill in the questionnaire by reading the sentences and then putting a ring around the answer which comes closest to how you feel. We realise that the sentences may not be exactly right for you, but please answer each question.

Consider the past month only.

1 I think I have lost confidence in myself

0	1	2	3	4
Not at all like me		A little like me		Exactly like me

2 I hate myself

0	1	2	3	4
Not at all like me		A little like me		Exactly like me

3 I am more short-tempered than I used to be

0	1	2	3	4
Not at all like me		A little like me		Exactly like me

4 I have begun to think that I am being punished

0	1	2	3	4
Not at all like me		A little like me		Exactly like me

5 I find it almost impossible to get any work done

0	1	2	3	4
Not at all like me		A little like me		Exactly like me

6 I regularly wake up hours earlier than I used to and can't get back to sleep

0	1	2	3	4
Not at all like me		A little like me		Exactly like me

7 I seem to have lost interest in things

0	1	2	3	4
Not at all like me		A little like me		Exactly like me

8 I feel that I am a total failure

0	1	2	3	4
Not at all like me		A little like me		Exactly like me

9 I have lost weight because I don't feel that I want to eat

0	1	2	3	4
Not at all like me		A little like me		Exactly like me

10 I feel that my mood is always lower in the morning

0	1	2	3	4
Not at all like me		A little like me		Exactly like me

Add your scores for the ten items

My total depression score is _____

Again, the higher the score the higher the level of depressive symptoms experienced. Your 'score' can be used for comparison with your score on the same questionnaire after you have spent some time trying out the techniques described and recommended in the book.

Note: It is very important to realise that if you do not have a high score on the checklist this does not necessarily mean you are not depressed, as such checklists cannot diagnose depression.

If you believe yourself to be depressed it is in your interests to go and talk to your family doctor who may wish to consider which treatment, if indicated, is most suitable for you.

What can you do to help yourself if you feel discouraged about the future or angry about the way that things have turned out?

Many of our patients say that they are angry but don't like to admit it. They say 'why me?', 'what have I done to deserve this?', or possibly they admit to feeling angry towards all of the people who don't have this problem. Indeed, it's not uncommon for them to feel very annoyed at the people who have tried to help: the doctors who can't find a cure, the friends and family who say that they understand, or that they are sorry for you and that it must be terrible to be like that. Sometimes it is just that every one else seems to be happy and to be able to get on with their lives.

We find that a particular problem for people with low mood is the great difficulty they have in getting themselves to do things.

They say that they find it difficult to get up in the morning, they say that they just want to stay in bed all day, not because they are tired, but because they can't face the day. It is often the case that they don't feel like preparing food for themselves or eating if someone else has made a meal for them.

So it isn't that the person with low mood has a pessimistic outlook that is often the main problem, it is often the problems which low mood cause in their lives that lead to the greatest distress to the individual and the family.

Chapter 4, 'Overcoming depression', provides guidelines for self-help. This chapter should be of interest and of value to all our readers, even those who don't regard themselves as being depressed, because two of the commonest reactions we have encountered to having tinnitus is to lose much of the motivation to do things, and an active avoidance of situations which were once potent sources of pleasure.

5 Analysing your tinnitus. The final section of this chapter is concerned with identifying the times and situations when your tinnitus is most troublesome and, the converse of this, the times and situations in which it is either absent or much less troublesome.

Some of our patients initially report that their tinnitus is always very loud, always a nuisance and always present. Most sufferers however, recognise that the loudness level and nuisance value fluctuate from time to time, sometimes apparently without reason. At other times it is clear that tinnitus is troublesome because of specific events or situations occurring. To gain insights into the variability or changes in your tinnitus experience it is necessary to monitor it.

There are two useful ways to tackle this. The first is to monitor your tinnitus in terms of its loudness and nuisance value over a number of days or weeks to determine possible trends. The second is a much more careful investigation of the possible 'triggers' or 'cues' that exist immediately prior to the onset of various levels of tinnitus loudness and nuisance value and the consequent effects of the tinnitus on you. We shall explain these approaches in more detail.

Monitoring trends. In this form of monitoring we shall ask you to rate your tinnitus in two ways. We want you to rate the loudness of the tinnitus sounds using the scale shown below.

We also want you to rate how much of a nuisance the tinnitus has been on that day, again using the scale shown below.

We recognise that loudness and nuisance or annoyance are related in that the louder the noise possibly the greater the annoyance. However, in a very recent study conducted in our department amongst a range of people with tinnitus, the relations between loudness and annoyance was very low. The study showed that loudness had little relationship with either patients' ability to tolerate tinnitus or their ratings of the severity of their tinnitus.

For **loudness:** rate your tinnitus loudness each day using a number between 0 and 6, where:

0   = tinnitus absent
1
2
3
4
5
6   = as loud as my tinnitus has ever been

For **nuisance:** rate your tinnitus overall each day in terms of how much of a nuisance, annoyance or interference it has been using a number between 0 and 6, where:

0   = not troublesome
1
2
3
4
5
6   = as troublesome as my tinnitus has ever been

You can make your ratings as often as you like each day but we would generally recommend a maximum of four times a day as our patients report that self-monitoring, in this way, leads you to pay more attention to your tinnitus, which is contrary to what we are recommending you do in later chapters of the book. In order for you to find a meaningful trend in the information you collect it is important to make your ratings at the same time each day. Rather like taking pills, it might be advisable to make each rating during a meal break. So, each day make your ratings during breakfast, lunch, tea and supper times.

Figure 2.1 Daily tinnitus ratings

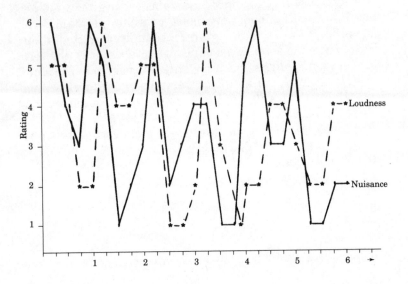

Make a record of your ratings on a chart as shown in Figure 2.1 by putting a point on the chart for both loudness and nuisance ratings, using different colours, and then join up the points as shown.

The example shown is with ratings drawn at random just to demonstate a completed chart for six days of recordings. The completed chart shown in Figure 2.2 is part of an actual chart kept by one of our patients.

What clues does the data collected by John give us about what might be making his tinnitus vary? Firstly, it is apparent that his loudness ratings are very high each evening (the fourth rating point each day). John later told us that he rarely went out in the evening and preferred to read or watch television. The loudness ratings are also quite high for most of the day on days 5 and 6. These days were weekend days when John was not working. Although he keeps himself quite busy on these days he admits that the activities are rarely those which require much effort of concentration.

Figure 2.2 John's daily tinnitus ratings

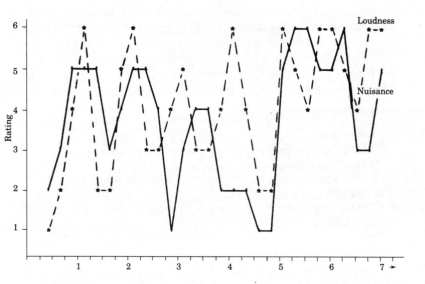

His nuisance ratings are quite high, particularly on days 5 and 6 (at the weekend), but also high on days 1 and 2. For much of the time, John's loudness and nuisance ratings are fairly similar. If John were to maintain his recordings over a few weeks it might be possible to discern some particular trends.

Are there particular times in the day or week when your tinnitus is particularly loud and of greater nuisance value? When is your tinnitus less of a problem? Can you relate changes in ratings to events that have happened? Are they related to the activities you have been engaged in, the people you were with or even the food that you ate?

Identification of triggers or cues to troublesome tinnitus. The previous method of monitoring your tinnitus is useful in identifying possible trends in the changes in loudness and nuisance value of your tinnitus over time. Although it may help you think about what may have caused the changes, you cannot be certain that your guesses are correct until you have checked your guesses. The best way to do this is using a daily tinnitus diary.

As with the previous method, it has the drawback of having you attend to your tinnitus but it will be of benefit.

All you have to do with this monitoring technique is once a day (perhaps first thing each morning) to spend some time thinking about how your tinnitus has been over the previous day. If there have been occasions when your tinnitus has been particularly bad, try to remember and make of note of the situation and conditions that existed for the half~hour before your noises were bad. Ask yourself (and answer) the following questions:

1 Where was I?   e.g. in the bedroom
2 What was I doing?   e.g. having a cup of tea in bed
3 How was I feeling?   e.g. very tired, low in mood
4 Who was I with?   e.g. no one but the cat
5 What time was it?
  What day/date was it? e.g. 9.15 a.m. on Tuesday 13th August

This list of questions is not meant to be an exhaustive list. You can add further questions which you believe might be relevant to your own individual case.

In Figure 2.3 we have shown an example of a tinnitus diary. The column heading can be varied to suit your particular needs. For example, you may wish to add ratings for nuisance or you may wish to record the times when you used your auditory masker. After keeping the daily diary for two or three weeks you will begin to see patterns emerge. In Chapter 6 we provide advice about how to make use of this information which is of course, specific to you and your situation.

You can continue to read the book chapter by chapter but may wish instead to go straight to the sections which deal with problems identified by you during this assessment chapter.

Chapter 3 looks at ways of overcoming anxiety, tension and worries, including anxiety provoked by particular situations.

Chapter 4 examines strategies for dealing effectively with depression. As with Chapter 3, the information contained can be worked through with specific reference to problems induced by tinnitus, but can also be used to tackle the problems which can arise independently of tinnitus but serve to make your tinnitus sounds much more difficult to live with.

Chapter 5 gives help with overcoming problems with sleeping.

Figure 2.3 Tinnitus diary

Day	Time	Where was I?	Doing what?	Loudness rating	With whom?	Feelings before

Chapter 6 relates to the work you did on monitoring your tinnitus. It is concerned with making changes in both your internal and external environment to overcome the effects of tinnitus.

Chapter 7 describes a technique we have been developing for use with tinnitus sufferers involving imagery, a technique that offers some exciting possibilities for coping with the condition.

At this point, return to the first page or two of this chapter. Are you going to put in the required effort to overcome your tinnitus? We hope so!

3 Overcoming anxiety

Chapter goals

By the end of this chapter we hope that you will achieve a number of goals. We expect that you will be able to:

1 Recognise and understand what anxiety is.
2 Appreciate the difference between anxiety which is helpful and anxiety which causes problems.
3 Understand the possible links between your tinnitus and anxiety.
4 Identify and try out a number of tried and tested effective strategies for overcoming anxiety.
5 Have some confidence that you can overcome any anxiety problems you may have and by so doing, improve the quality of your life.

Tackling and overcoming anxiety are essential steps in overcoming tinnitus distress.

This chapter has been designed as a guide to show you how to effectively overcome any anxiety problems you may have. Please do not be put off by the term 'anxiety'.

You may not regard yourself as anxious, but nevertheless, we hope that you will find the information and advice of interest and useful. We have chosen to write about anxiety because it is a very common problem. It has been variously estimated that 1 in 10 people will consult their general practitioner on some occasion for help with anxiety. The problem is thought to be even more common in people with severe tinnitus.

The chapter is divided into three sections:

1 What is anxiety? This section explains what is meant by anxiety, its causes and effects.

2 How to control anxiety. This part examines ways of controlling and overcoming the symptoms of anxiety by using relaxation techniques, distraction, control of distressing thoughts and instructions for dealing with panic.

3 Managing avoidance. How to manage the problem of avoidance and how to rebuild your confidence.

What is anxiety?

We are all familiar with a long list of words, all of which essentially refer to the same or similar state we shall call 'anxiety'. Such a list would include tension, nervousness, panic, fear, apprehension, uncertainty, and so on.

Anxiety affects people in three closely related ways:

Firstly, we experience physical or somatic symptoms of anxiety - the things that happen to your body when you are anxious.

Secondly, we experience psychological or cognitive symptoms - the thoughts and feelings we have when anxious.

Thirdly, we behave differently when anxious; this component of anxiety is concerned with what we actually do.

Let's look at some examples of what we mean. The lists that follow are by no means exhaustive lists of signs and symptoms. You will probably not experience all of these and there may be some others that you experience that we have not included. Bear in mind too that we can experience these to varying degrees of intensity, they may last for varying amounts of time and vary in how often they occur.

The **physical** symptoms may include:

muscle tension
headache or feelings of pressure in the head
heart racing, palpitations
feeling hot, excessive perspiration
dizziness
shakiness of hands, limbs or body
tingling sensations
dry mouth, swallowing difficulties
'butterflies' in your stomach
blurred vision
a desire to go to the toilet
weak legs
breathing difficulties, chest tightness, rapid breathing.

The **psychological** symptoms may include:

thinking that you might die
thinking that you may lose control
feeling frightened, panicky
worrying that you may pass out
worrying that you might vomit

worrying that people will notice you
feeling that you need to escape or run away
worrying that you might have a heart attack or fit
thinking there is something wrong with your mind or brain
thinking that you are losing your mind.

The **behavioural** symptoms may include:

making excuses to avoid doing something or going somewhere
leaving places before you planned to or ought to
avoiding going out alone
using taxis rather than buses or trains
only shopping when it's quiet
having your hair done at home rather than face the salon
using alcohol or tranquillisers to enable you to cope
crossing the street to avoid having to meet people
not answering your door or telephone
not talking in social gatherings.

Let's now look at anxiety more closely so that you will be able to understand how and why your symptoms occur.

The most surprising thing to many people is to be told that **anxiety is a normal healthy reaction**. It is Nature's way of equipping us to cope with threats and dangers.

Imagine yourself crossing a busy road. Suddenly, you hear a car's brakes screech and a loud car horn. You will almost certainly jump or run off the road, even before you have had time to think or even look to see whether it is you who is in danger. When you get to the pavement you will be left feeling shaky, your heart will be racing, and you may experience some of the signs and symptoms of physical anxiety listed above. What has happened to your body?

Your ears have picked up the sounds of the car's horn and brakes, and your brain has recognised that there is some kind of danger and switched on an anxiety response. It has happened without you being conscious about deciding what best to do. It has happened automatically. Your inbuilt 'responding to danger' system has saved you.

The anxiety response allows your brain to quickly send signals to all parts of your body, so allowing you to escape from danger. Chemical messages are sent to your heart to speed it up. This means that it can pump blood more rapidly. To make this clear we can look at the effect on the muscles of your legs. The anxiety response allows them to develop sufficient tone to enable them to work quickly to take you away from the threat.

You breathe more quickly, so that your heart has enough oxygen to work harder. This is because, if your muscles are to work harder, they have to have enough oxygen-rich blood. As your body gives more blood to your limbs, your stomach (and other organs) become relatively deprived of blood. This is, of course, a perfectly natural and safe process, however, it may trigger off sensations of stomach-churning or 'butterflies'. Your brain, too, becomes relatively depleted of oxygen (again nothing to worry about) and sometimes lightheadedness or dizziness may ensue. At the same time (because of the increased blood flow to your muscles), your skin may become warmer, so that you may notice that you have begun to perspire, as a way of helping to cool your skin.

The anxiety response is automatic. It serves to enable your body to either 'fight' the threat or run away: the so called 'fight or flight' response.

Moderate amounts of anxiety can improve our performance in a range of situations. An actor who did not get 'keyed up' for a performance or a student who did not feel some urgency before an exam could not expect to perform at her best. Have you ever watched weight lifters before they try to lift a great weight? They go to enormous lengths to 'psych' themselves up and will look as if they are intending to fight someone or themselves. This allows them to perform at an optimum level. In some situations if you are too relaxed, your performance will suffer. On the other hand, as we all know, if you are too anxious your performance suffers too, and what we all wish is to maintain an optimum level of anxiety.

The psychological symptoms of anxiety listed earlier in this chapter are mainly about being fearful or apprehensive about something that might happen. Sometimes it is about a specific possible outcome: 'I might have a heart attack' or 'I will go mad', but occasionally it may not be specific. Sometimes we have a vague feeling of impending doom. Sometimes fear can be useful because it can help us become more motivated to do something about a possible threat. For example, if you feel fearful of an impending exam it may encourage you to put a bit more time and effort into revising and hence equip you better to face the exam threat.

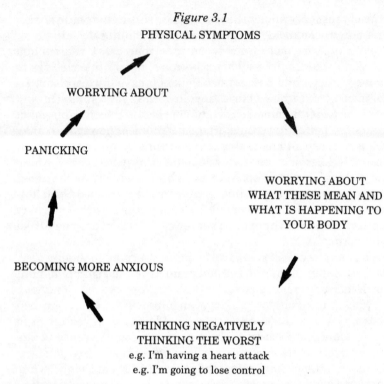

Figure 3.1
PHYSICAL SYMPTOMS

WORRYING ABOUT

PANICKING

WORRYING ABOUT
WHAT THESE MEAN AND
WHAT IS HAPPENING TO
YOUR BODY

BECOMING MORE ANXIOUS

THINKING NEGATIVELY
THINKING THE WORST
e.g. I'm having a heart attack
e.g. I'm going to lose control

Sometimes, however, anxious thoughts are unpleasant hindrances. Too many thoughts, or thoughts that are high in anxiety will interfere with normal thinking, will disrupt concentration and may lead to a state of chronic tension or worrying.

Physical symptoms of anxiety are often accompanied by thinking about and interpreting the bodily sensations. If you don't understand what is happening to your body and why it is reacting as it is you will try to find an explanation. Sometimes you reach negative conclusions: 'I am going mad'; 'I am losing control'; 'I have something seriously wrong with my body.' These kinds of inaccurate thoughts or explanations will only serve to fuel the anxiety and make it worse.

You begin to establish a vicious circle as shown in Figure 3.1. The physical symptoms of anxiety are switched on by an automatic anxiety response which has evolved to help us prepare to deal with threats. This automatic response may be readily triggered in some individuals and, as we have seen, may occur in the absence of threat. Feeling frightened is a natural and normal part of the anxiety response. However, the negative thoughts that arise, such as "I'm going to make a fool of myself", will tend to make the anxiety symptoms worse by adding fuel to the anxiety. Over time, negative thinking can induce the anxiety response with its accompanying physical symptoms.

The third component of anxiety is your behaviour when anxious. The common and understandable response is to avoid situations which might trigger the anxiety response, thus trying to avoid becoming very anxious. Whilst this may stop you feeling anxious in the short term it can lead to a serious deterioration in your ability to go to certain places or do particular things that in the past were not a problem. By avoiding situations you, in effect, ensure that you cannot rid yourself of anxiety problems. You deny yourself the opportunity of making progress. Another behaviour indicative of anxiety within situations is leaving them prematurely. Escaping, like avoiding, has a powerful reinforcing or rewarding quality about it (because you are escaping from anxiety), but this too prolongs any anxiety problem you may have.

Anxiety may become a problem when it occurs on occasions when there is no danger or when it continues long after the threat is past. Feeling your body preparing itself for 'flight or fight' in the absence of danger can be both unpleasant and a disadvantage because it begins to interfere with your life.

What causes anxiety problems? Most of our patients who have anxiety problems ask why symptoms begin. There is rarely a single answer to this question because for most people there are several factors which have played a part.

Some people are born with a predisposition or vulnerability to becoming anxious. They have a nervous system which reacts very easily to pressures and threats. Research has shown that for such individuals their nervous system reacts more readily and often more intensively when they are tired or under stress. When such persons subsequently develop tinnitus it is not at all surprising that they should become more tense and anxious.

For others who are born with a more hardy nervous system, anxiety problems can develop following a very wide range of problems and events. Indeed, a considerable body of research has shown how your likelihood of becoming ill is related to the kinds of life events you have experienced in a particular period of time.

The best known work of this kind was carried out by Holmes and Rahe and published in a scientific journal more than 20 years ago. They constructed a list of events which from their research were known to be sources of significant pressure on individuals. They then put these into a rank order (from the most to the least stressful) and gave each event a score to indicate its importance as a 'stressor'. The event found to be most stressful was 'death of spouse'; they gave this a score of 100. Next came 'divorce', 73; 'marital separation', 65; 'imprisonment', 63; 'death of a close family member', 63; and so on. For tinnitus sufferers, the most appropriate item on the scale is 'personal injury or illness' with a score of 53. The scale also identified a large number of items concerned with change, e.g. 'change in recreation'. This strongly suggests that, for tinnitus sufferers, changes in many areas of life (such as avoiding certain places) adds to the life events stress score. Holmes and Rahe used the total life events score to predict the likelihood of illness. The higher the score, the greater the chance of becoming ill.

The previous paragraphs looking at the causes of anxiety problems looked at inherited vulnerability and how stressful life events contributed to its development. We now want to address the subject of how your thoughts can increase anxiety. We are not really suggesting this as a cause but as a potent explanation of why anxiety problems can grow and be maintained.

Suppose you are sleeping alone in a hotel room in the middle of New York, and are woken in the middle of the night by a loud noise. You sit up quickly and become immediately aware of your heart thumping in your chest. Remember that this reaction is the automatic anxiety response, preparing you to deal with the 'threat' by 'fight or flight'. The reaction occurs before you have time to think and take stock of the situation. Your first thought might be 'someone must have broken into my room'. If this is your thought then you will feel even more frightened, and no doubt become aware of many of the physical and psychological symptoms listed earlier. However, if your thoughts are 'I must have left the window ajar and as it's a very windy night it must have banged shut' then your automatic anxiety response will start to slow down and stop. Your symptoms of fear will subside and you will settle down again to sleep.

When you begin to notice your tinnitus what goes through your mind? Take a few seconds to close your eyes and allow your mind to wonder ...

Did you notice that you began to become tense?

Did the problems that you thought had been put to the back of your mind start to cause distress?

If you sometimes have difficulty falling asleep, did you notice that the thoughts which tend to keep you awake were similar to those that just came in to your mind?

Did you notice that the more that you concentrated on the upsetting thoughts, the more tense you became?

Did you find it quite difficult to think of anything else when thoughts of tinnitus occupied your mind?

This checklist contains many of the problems which many of our patients have been troubled by. This isn't a complete list, so some of your difficulties may not be included. However, we hope that you will be able to recognise at least some of the most troubling results of anxiety.

Read each statement and put a tick in the box of those which give an idea of your feelings.

1 Pain or discomfort in your muscles ☐
2 A feeling of shakiness in your body ☐
3 Excessive perspiration ☐
4 Noticing that your mouth seems to be unusually dry ☐
5 Noticing that you seem to have episodes of
   breathing more rapidly than usual ☐
6 Noticing that your heart seems to have been
   (i) beating more quickly than usual ☐
   (ii) giving you 'palpitations' ☐
7 A slight feeling of choking ☐
8 Slight feeling of dizziness or faintness ☐
9 Feeling that your muscles are tense and uncomfortable ☐
10 Having discomfort (butterflies) in your stomach ☐
11 Noticing that you seem to be
   (i) tired more often than usual ☐
   (ii) more easily exhausted than usual ☐
12 Thinking that you may criticised by others ☐
13 Noticing that you are more 'jumpy' than usual ☐
14 Thinking that the fear which you sometimes notice
   means that you are going mad ☐
15 Feeling that you want to try and run away from
   situations which didn't used to bother you ☐

16 Finding that you have begun to worry that you
might 'pass out' in situations that cause you to
become anxious ☐

17 Finding that you often think that some thing terrible
is about to happen ☐

18 Finding it difficult to maintain your concentration ☐

19 A feeling of being apprehensive in situations that
didn't used to be so much of a problem ☐

20 Noticing that you have begun to worry about
minor physical sensations (e.g. tingling or pins
and needles) more often than usual ☐

21 Thinking that you seem to be 'at a distance' from
what is going on in social situations ☐

22 Finding that you are generally more apprehensive
than you used to be ☐

23 Finding that you have begun to rearrange the times
that you go shopping to try and avoid becoming anxious ☐

24 Finding that you have begun to take tablets to calm down ☐

25 Finding that you have started to drink more than you
used to ☐

26 Noticing that you have fewer social activities because
you worry about going to them ☐

27 Finding that you have come to require some one to be
with you in social situations ☐

28 Finding that you are more 'accident prone' than you
used to be ☐

29 Finding that you are making more mistakes than normal ☐

30 Finding that you are going to your doctors for reassurance
rather than for treatment ☐

31 Finding that it takes you longer to go to sleep ☐

Note Many of these feelings may be the result of physical
difficulties which have produced the hearing problems or tinnitus.
Therefore, make sure that you have spoken to your doctor about
this and understand which problems are caused by anxiety.

How to control anxiety

Tried and tested strategies for overcoming anxiety

As we said in the introduction, anxiety has three aspects:
(a) The physical sensations
(b) The psychological problems
(c) The altered lifestyle.

Therefore, when seeking ways of reducing your anxiety we can use each of the above as a guide.

To find out which of these you believed is the most important, follow the scoring instructions.

Scoring instuctions

The answer sheet is divided into three sections. Each of questions which you have just answered fell into one of categories that we discussed above. You were asked about of three things:

(a) Physical sensations
(b) Psychological difficulties
(c) Changes in the way that you live

1 Look again at your results.

2 Find the number of questions in each section which you said was true for you and put the total in the box below:

(a) Physical sensation: questions 1 to 11 ☐
(b) Psychological difficulties: questions 12 to 22 ☐
(c) Changes in the way that you live: questions 23 to 31 ☐

3 Turn to the section which seems to be the most important for you in the 'Suggested help list'.

Note Some of the difficulties listed above can be the result of the physical problems which caused the tinnitus. Therefore, if you you are not sure if your problems are the result of anxiety seek the advice of your doctor.

It is obviously better to concentrate on overcoming those problems which seem to be the result of anxiety. Although we realise that some patients are most distressed by their physical problems. If you fall into this category we don't mean that you 'accept defeat'. We hope that you will be able to use the strategies in the chapter to reduce the distress which the problems cause to an absolute minimum.

Suggested help list

Physical sensations of anxiety. As a result of the way in which the human body has evolved, we react to anxiety in predictable ways. The problem is that while this set of reactions was appropriate to the lifestyle of our ancestors, it can cause problems today.

When we are under stress the rate of breathing increases, this may not seem to be of great interest until you realise that the effects can be:

Feelings of shakiness in your body
Rapid heartbeat or 'palpitations'
A slight choking sensation
A feeling of faintness
A feeling of 'pins and needles'

When you notice that you are breathing more quickly than usual:

(a) Stop whatever you are doing if it is safe and convenient to do so

(b) Slow your breathing down. Remember, the rate you need is the normal rate so don't try to take abnormally large and 'forced' breaths

(c) Focus your mind on to the breaths

(d) Notice that the rate is responsive and it will slow down if you allow it to do so

(e) If you find it helpful, cup your hands loosely over your mouth and nose. Begin to breathe slowly out from your mouth and in through your nose

(f) It may also be a good idea to take some time to notice your normal rate of breathing so that you will have this as a target when you are overbreathing

We often find that many of our patients (not just those with tinnitus) have a great deal of muscular tension. However, they often don't realise this. They will often take a great deal of convincing that the pain and discomfort that they feel can be the result of anxiety. The most powerful demonstration that this is indeed the case comes after they have regularly practiced a programme of relaxation exercises.

The relaxation exercises can be found at the end of the book. However, before you begin to use them think.

If you find that your tinnitus causes you greater problems when you are sitting quietly with nothing to occupy your mind, it may not be a good idea to spend time relaxing! A more helpful strategy would be to find ways to deal with the upsetting thoughts (see the next section) and then to use the relaxation. Try not to make the mistake of becoming anxious about not being relaxed!

Managing avoidance

Psychological difficulties. The response to anxiety can be thought of as similar to that of a fire alarm. When it is triggered, all of the systems which it controls come into action at once. The result can be that the alarm works correctly and a possibly disastrous fire is safely extinguished with the minimum of damage. However, if the system reacts inappropriately (for example, to the smoke from a lighted cigarette in an ashtray) then the damage caused by the sprinklers will be out of proportion to the threat of fire.

When you notice that your heart is racing, your mouth dry and your perspiration in danger of becoming an embarrassment, it is a reasonable assumption that you are anxious.

Why do you think that we could make this guess from so little evidence?

The explanation is this: many of the reactions to anxiety occur in other situations but are not noticed to the same degree. Think about how your body would react to running a race. The increased heart rate and perspiration, would be accepted as normal. Therefore, you would be less likely to worry about them and so allow your body to come back into its normal balance.

The problems which the anxiety reaction causes are not only the result of our 'stone age' bodies. In addition, the causes of anxiety have changed from immediate threats to persistent pressures. The worry about tinnitus is a good example. The sufferer has the problem in the back of their mind at all times; even sleep is disturbed. The person has the problems of fatigue, in addition to the corrosive effects of continual bodily reactions to anxiety.

Most people who say this under these circumstances seem to mean that they are having to struggle with problems that they have never had before. The main source of worry is fear of the future. The course of physical problems can be gauged from consultations with medical practitioners. The psychological aspect is one you can help yourself with; the more that you understand about the reasons for your anxiety the less frightening it will seem. The future may seem very black at the moment, but it is seldom as bad as the worst fears, nor as good as we would wish.

When you begin to notice your tinnitus, what goes through

your mind? Take a few seconds to close your eyes and allow your mind to wonder ...

Did you notice that you began to become tense?

Did the problems that you thought had been put to the back of your mind start to cause distress?

If you sometimes have difficulty falling asleep, did you notice that the thoughts which tend to keep you awake were similar to those that just came in to your mind?

Did you notice that the more that you concentrated on the upsetting thoughts, the more tense you became?

Did you find it quite difficult to think of anything else when thoughts of tinnitus occupied your mind?

The majority of our anxious patients say that they find themselves becoming tense when they don't have anything to occupy their mind. They also say that they notice thoughts that usually only become a problem late at night. The 'problem-causing thoughts' are more easily dismissed during the day.

Thinking that problems will occur
This is obviously not a problem in itself; it doesn't seem possible to live a life without at least some problems. The point is, are your worries:

(a) excessive

(b) based on an accurate picture of the situation

(c) about subjects that you can actually change for the better.

The best way to tackle these problems is to take 'a second look'. This is best done by writing the problems down. Take a sheet of paper and put a line from top to bottom; write 'problem' on the left side and 'evidence' on the right hand side. Then fold the paper along the line and write your list of problems. Take some time; try to make the list as complete as possible. When you have done this, go through the list and cross out all of the problems that you cannot do anything about. By all means come back to them later, but recognise that you can't do anything about them. Also put a line through those which now seem to be trivial. Unfold the piece of paper and by the side of the problems which are left write down the evidence that:

(a) the problem is as large as you thought

(b) the problem is as black and white as you think it is

Leave a space underneath each piece of 'evidence'. Put the paper away for an hour or two then come back to it with a fresh mind.

The evidence may not seem as convincing as before, but if you are still convinced by it, spend some time trying to challenge it. A helpful way to do so is to imagine that you are a lawyer trying to find out the truth about the evidence. How would you do it? For example, would you believe it just because you have heard it once? Or would you look for evidence of your own which would contradict it and support your case? Most lawyers would do the second of these, so how will you do it? Use these guidelines:

(a) Try to find any 'absolutes', i.e. I always or You never, etc. To disprove this is relatively simple, you only have to find one example in the opposite direction, so think carefully.

(b) Do other people tend to share your view? It doesn't mean you are wrong if they don't, but it may by a good idea to find out why.

(c) Is this a view that you have held for some time? It may have been reasonable at that time but have things changed?

Write down the contradictory evidence. How does the problem seem now? In order to make your point will you have to use more moderate language? How many of the original problems on the list are left? We sometimes hear our patients say that although they have reduced the list by a substantial number, it is only the simple or unimportant problems that have gone. The best way to find out if this is the case for you is to write that down on the list and work through it as we have just outlined. They often find that although some important problems remain, others have been dealt with, and that several of those which remain have been altered, so that they can be more easily coped with.

When people complain of poor concentration, the problem is often that they are concentrating, but not on the subject in hand. This seems to be the difficulty of some patients with tinnitus. They become haunted by the sound; it seems to attract their attention away from other things.

In other cases, the sufferer has a 'spiral of distress' in which:

(a) they worry about their noise,

(b) and so concentrate upon it,

(c) this causes more anxiety,

(d) with the result that they worry about the effects of anxiety,

(e) this gives the impression that they are 'getting worse'

(f) the sufferer becomes anxious and so more conscious of their tinnitus.

The sufferer becomes increasingly distressed, often complaining of poor concentration.

In some cases, the sufferer's mood can be a significant contribution to their poor concentration. As you can see from the 'spiral of distress', the effect of worry can be more worry and so more distress. When worry becomes a constant, unwelcome companion, life will sometimes become little more than a chore. This will cause lower mood (see Chapter 4), a consequence of which is that even thinking requires more effort than usual.

The most obvious answers often seem to be the most obscure, until we realise what they are. This is true of problems with concentration. When tinnitus happens, in addition to all of the unpleasant 'psychological' consequences, hearing is often impaired. As we have said, this is obvious, but sometimes sufferers don't want to admit this to others, or on occasion, to themselves. They are anxious that their hearing impairment isn't noticed, so they give the impression that their attention has wandered off the subject.

The paragraphs above may have given the impression that only one cause for poor concentration will be found. This tends not to be the case. Therefore, if you find that you are having difficulty in concentrating, ask the following questions:

(a) am I low in mood?

(b) am I tending to concentrate on my tinnitus, rather than the matter at hand

(c) am I in the 'spiral of distress'?

(d) is it simply that I am missing the thread of conversations because of the tinnitus noise?

Keep a record of when the problem occurs.

	What I was doing	How I felt
Monday		
Tuesday		
Wednesday		
Thursday		

Friday

Saturday

Sunday

Self-confidence

We find that many of our patients could do a great deal to help themselves become less anxious. Indeed, they have lots of good ideas about the sort of things which would be helpful.
– The problem isn't that they don't know what to do.
– The problem isn't that their ideas are too ambitious or impractical.

For many people it seems to be that the anxiety generated by their fear of tinnitus has robbed them of their self-confidence. They have the feeling that what they are able to do won't be enough to make a difference. We hope that after working through the following suggestions you will see yourself in a more realistic and a more positive light.

We often ask our patients to put into words:

1 The way that they see themselves **now**
2 How they would **like to be**.

This exercise is reproduced below so that you can complete it for yourself. Write down one word which describes you by each number. It isn't essential to fill in all of the numbers or to have the same number in each column. However, take some time to think about the words and try to put as good a description as you can.

Write one word which describes you by each number.

Words that describe me now	Words that describe how I would like to be
1	1
2	2
3	3
4	4
5	5
6	6
7	7
8	8

After our patients have completed their lists, we ask them to go back through it and note if the words that they have used about themselves have been:

(a) **Good**, i.e. positive, helpful, optimistic, pleasant. If this is correct then put + by the word.

(b) **Neutral**, i.e. ordinary, not pleasant or unpleasant, easily overlooked or forgotten. If this is correct then put 0 by the word.

(c) **Bad**, i.e. negative, pessimistic, unpleasant. If this is correct then put - by the word.

When you have completed this, count up the numbers of **good, neutral** and **bad** descriptions. Write the number of each in the boxes below:

Words that describe me now   Words that describe how
I would like to be

+ ☐   + ☐
0 ☐   0 ☐
– ☐   – ☐

Ask yourself some questions about what you have written:

– Have you written an equal number of good and bad descriptions?

– Are the words which describe you now and those which describe how you wish to be equally balanced?

We find that most of our patients have more negatives in the first column than the second. This is a reflection of the dissatisfaction which they feel with themselves. The self that they would like to become is sometimes just a mirror image of the way that they see themselves at present.

It is sometimes the case that we are often able to offer criticism of ourselves that would provoke anger if another person tried to use similar words. If this is the case, why do we believe that 'it must be true because I have said it'? At least in part, it seems to be because we don't take the time to 'think through' the thoughts which cause us to become upset.

When we get upset it is almost the case that we think that the upsetting thought must have been true because it made us upset! Does this seem to be a helpful way to think about yourself and your problems?

We think that it is very important to look for some evidence to question your views and put them into perspective. This allows you the time to regain a sense of control over the problems and helps to make you more confident about solving them. As we have said before, this does not mean 'the perfect solution', just one which offers some hope of improvement. Bearing this in mind, look again at the numbers of **good** and **bad** scores which you have. The most usual pattern is, as we said, a larger number of negatives in the 'as I am now' column. If you find that this isn't the case for you, **congratulations** - you can go to the end of the chapter. However, if you are like the majority of us, read on ...

Why do you think that you have this result? The most obvious answer is that this is 'how it is', in other words, the answers are a true reflection of your life. Look back over the list; one thing that is missing is any idea of how true the answers are. As you can understand, a - may not cause many problems if it is only a minor criticism that happens occasionally. Therefore, rather than accepting that this may be the case for you, go back to the word list and show how much you believe that the word is generally true of you. The easiest way to do this is to put a number between 1 and 10, i.e., if it is only a minor criticism then give it 1, if it is a significant problem then rate it 10. Obviously, if it is in between then give it an appropriate number.

When you have done this, look again at the words; they may still describe you. However, when you rated them did you notice that the problem was given a lower number after you had thought about it? We sometimes find that this is very helpful to some patients; they feel that the problems seem somehow less threatening.

The idea of rating your problems can be a powerful way of helping yourself to overcome the problems which give rise to the anxiety. Therefore, when you notice yourself becoming anxious, go through the process we have just used.

1 Notice that you are getting anxious.
2 Organise your thoughts and write them down.
3 Rate the thoughts 1 to 10.
4 Think of how to change the problem thoughts.
5 Have the courage to put the changes into effect.

Changes in the way you live. You may wish that the tinnitus would simply disappear overnight. This is of course the best solution; however, distinguish between dreams of perfection and the everyday work required to make life worth living. The wish

Table 3.1 Daily diary

	Morning	Afternoon	Night
Monday			
Tuesday			
Wednesday			
Thursday			
Friday			
Saturday			
Sunday			

for magic may become the barrier which prevents you from making any improvement to your life. This is one reason why it is so important to try to think through all of the possible causes for the unpleasant feelings that you notice. A rule of thumb is:

'if the reason for your problem is obvious, and you can put it into effect at once without any effort, it is likely that you haven't got the right reason'

– Set targets for yourself that are achievable; accept that you may not be able to do all that you would wish as quickly you used to.

– However, this does not mean that you can't do anything.

– Take the time to plan your day (use the Daily diary in Table 3.1)

– See if you can include a 'treat' for yourself.

– When you have written down the daily routine, put a star by those things that you do because you choose to.

– Remember, the basic domestic chores are things which have to be done whether you enjoy them or not.

– Include things to do which you have chosen to do **but do something each day**.

– Take things easily, go at a sensible pace.

– **Remember**, sitting down wishing and worrying will not help in the long term.

To recap, what we are saying is:

(a) That if we asked you to give a list of your problems, you would be able to give a complete account of the number. However, we would be surprised if the size of each of them was as great as you may think at the moment.

(b) That it is very difficult to get a problem 'down to size' by letting it run through your mind. Indeed, it is often the case that problems get larger the more that you think about them.

(c) That many people who think that they have a problem with anxiety don't. The problem is that they have not:

(i) found out exactly what are the thoughts which are making them anxious.

(ii) tried to find out if the fear that they have is reasonable or is it the worst possible case which rarely happens.

(d) That the fears can be most quickly put into a manageable size by taking sensible steps to challenge the problem thoughts, i.e.

(i) looking for evidence which would help them to decide

if the 'problem thoughts' are reasonable.

      (ii) putting the more reasonable thoughts into effect.

  (e) Remember the short title of the programme **NORTH** (see above).

The effect of anxiety can be to make you lose confidence in yourself. This sometimes means that you become frightened of situations which did not previously cause problems. This is not unusual; many tinnitus sufferers have similar problems. The British Tinnitus Association (see the 'Useful addresses' section towards the end of the book) will provide support and help you to to learn more about the condition.

4 Overcoming depression

Chapter goals

By the end of this chapter we hope that you will be able to notice if there is a link between your mood and the problems in your life, including tinnitus. In addition, you will perhaps know yourself a little better and so feel more confident that you can begin to take a different view of your situation and so allow your mood to lift.

We also think that it is important for you to understand the different ways in which the word 'depression' can be used. It can mean that the person will need to speak to their doctor and may need tablets as part of their treatment. However, it can also be used to show that 'things hadn't been going too well' or 'I'm discouraged' or simply 'I'm feeling fed up'. Therefore, 'depression' isn't an all or nothing label; rather, it is a broad description of a variety of feelings.

Since you began to notice your tinnitus, has your mood changed? What can you do to help yourself if you feel discouraged about the future or angry about the way that things have turned out? Many of our patients say that they are angry but don't like to admit it. They say 'Why me?', 'What have I done to deserve this?', or possibly they admit to feeling angry towards all of the people who don't have this problem.

Indeed, it's not uncommon for them to feel very annoyed at the people who have tried to help:
– the doctors who can't find a cure
– the friends and family who say that they understand or that they are sorry for you
– sometimes it is just that every one else seems to be happy and to be able to get on with their lives.

How would you describe your mood? The following list of words contains some which people have said describe their depression.
– Read through the words
– Find those which seem to describe you

– Write a capital letter 'D' in the box on the right.

1	Low	☐	**2**	Sad	☐
3	Miserable	☐	**4**	Fed up	☐
5	Hopeless	☐	**6**	Dejected	☐
7	Unhappy	☐	**8**	Lethargy	☐

When you looked back over your responses, did you find that your mood was lower than you thought? We find that many patients don't realise how low they feel until they are asked to think about it. However, remember: a score on a short question-naire does not take the place of a diagnosis! **If you believe that your mood is low (for whatever reason) get an appointment with your doctor and ask for their advice.**

When we try to help people to fight their low mood they some-times believe that they can't do anything. The reason that they give is that their mood is just a reflection of 'the way that life has treated them'. The problems which they have, e.g. tinnitus, are real enough so they say 'what can they do to change them?'

What we hope to do is to show you that, although your mood may be low for good reason, what you do can make a difference; your mood may not have to be as low as it has become. We can't aim to remove the cause of sadness, distress or disease, it would be a silly claim for anyone to make. However, does that have to mean that no progress is possible and that any attempt is going to be futile and so not worth the effort? If that is your view (and many of our patients used to share it), can you be sure unless you are willing to put the evidence for it to the test?

The point isn't that you will be wrong, but it is often helpful to look again (even at circumstances that you know well) to see if there have been any changes that have yet to be noticed. Think about how you would feel in the following situations, then put a number which represents your view into the box on the right.

Very happy		Happy		OK		Unhappy	Very unhappy
1	2	3	4	5	6	7	8	9

1	Winning a large amount of money	☐
2	Losing a large amount of money	☐
3	Becoming unemployed	☐
4	Learning of the death of a close friend	☐
5	Falling in love	☐
6	Going on holiday	☐
7	Having to do the washing up after a large meal	☐

We hope that the list has a range of numbers. Some of the incidents are generally regarded as pleasant, others less so. However, if you read through the list again, **for some questions** it should be possible to find emotions dissimilar to those which you have written.

The item about going on holiday, for example, must depend on when, where, how and with whom you make the trip. The third question, again, can only be answered when more information is provided. The difference in the emotional impact of:

(a) Planned retirement with a good pension
and
(b) being fired without a reference because of theft
could well be substantial.

We find that a particular problem for people with low mood is the great difficulty they have in setting themselves to do things. They say that they find it difficult to get up in the morning; they say that they just want to stay in bed all day, not because they are tired, but because they can't face the day. It is often the case that they don't feel like preparing food for themselves or eating if someone else has made a meal for them.

So it often isn't the person's low mood which is the main problem. It can be the case that their greatest cause of sadness is the problems in their lives which their low mood has caused. This is difficult for many of our patients to accept, but remember, we are not saying that low mood isn't a problem. The point is that low mood is not the full picture. Things are often difficult, but does that mean that you can't do anything to improve your situation? The message of this chapter and the entire book is that you can make a difference! We hope that you will soon have the skills which you may need and the confidence to use them.

To help you to get a wider view of your situation, fill in the following checklist by putting a tick in the box on the right:

1 The low mood began shortly after my tinnitus, so the tinnitus must have caused it ☐
2 If I could only wake up one morning without my tinnitus then I would be OK ☐
3 The tinnitus makes everything impossible; I can't get any pleasure out of life as long as the tinnitus is a problem ☐
4 The low mood has made everything impossible; I can only get any pleasure out of life when the low mood has gone ☐
5 As long as I have tinnitus the low mood will remain;

I can't do anything to shake it off ☐

6 I have never had low mood before, so I don't think
that it will be possible for me to challenge the problems
that it causes ☐

7 I think that the low mood or the tinnitus are a curse and
that it is unfair that it should happen to me ☐

8 I don't think that anyone could deal with the problems
that I have ☐

9 Whenever I notice the tinnitus I find that my mood
goes down ☐

10 I don't think that any one else understands the
problems that tinnitus causes to sufferers ☐

11 I think that it just isn't possible to stop myself from
becoming depressed if something unpleasant happens
to me ☐

12 I think that if my mood becomes depressed it is
the result of things that I can't control ☐

13 Because tinnitus is a barrier when talking to others
I am going to be an isolated and unhappy person ☐

14 If I ever make a mistake because of my tinnitus I should
feel upset or ashamed of myself ☐

15 I think it is always appropriate to become frustrated
if I find that I am not able to do as I wish ☐

16 If members of my family or friends seem to have
lost patience with me since the tinnitus began,
then there must be something wrong with me. ☐

The first point to make is that many people complain that the statements didn't cover all of their problems. This is obviously true, but we find that most people feel that at least some of their greatest difficulties have been covered. The list is only intended to give you somewhere to begin to look again at the possible causes of your low mood.

We hope that as you work through the chapter you will find the difficulties which we didn't put into the list less troublesome than before. So you will be able to use the skills which you have to tackle many different problems whether or not they are related to low mood or tinnitus.

Ways to recognise the problem thoughts that will tend to contribute to your low mood

1 Can you find any **absolutes** in the ways that you are thinking about some important problems?

Absolutes include the following words
- Always
- Never
- Everyone
- Perfect
- Must

2 Are you mind-reading?
- Mind-reading is often very difficult to spot, because we all tend to do it from time to time. Therefore, it is often easier to see it in others than ourselves. Try to notice the occasions that you hear others say that they 'know' the reason that X did this or that. However, try to see if there can be another reason that the person acted as they did. Is it true that the only reason that people do this is because they are thinking ...

3 Are you setting yourself a set of circumstances in which it isn't possible to win?
- The easiest way to find out if this is true for you, is to notice how often you think that you have failed each day. Make a note of how many times you use the words
  - Should
  - Ought

4 Are you setting yourself further problems by seeing yourself and your problems as a diagnosis?
- The disadvantages of concentrating on the diagnosis (tinnitus) are
- How the tinnitus actually affects you depends not only upon your physical status, but also on what sort of person you are and how you react to the problems that it presents.
- The diagnosis often doesn't give an indication of how the physical problems (if any) will progress.

5 Are you crystal ball gazing?
- The future may seem to be following a particular path; try to notice the times that you make predictions about how things will turn out.

6 Are you using the **mental magnifying glass**?
– The mental magnifying glass tends to be used to
   – Seek out problems that might otherwise have been missed.
   – Make problems that would be difficult to solve, seem so large that they are overwhelming.

7 Are you always playing the **rejection record**?
Do you find that you are always criticising yourself or other people?

Record problem thoughts

The problem thoughts tend to make your mood lower than it would otherwise be. Use the help sheets to show you the relationship between your thoughts and your mood. We find that, in general, the more that our patients understand about this, the more confident they feel when trying to lift their low mood. The first thing that you will need to do is become familiar with the process of 'thinking about your thoughts'. Many people find this very difficult, so don't expect to get it right the first time; give yourself time to learn this new skill.

First help sheet

Each day write down the **problem thoughts** as soon as you notice them:
   – They will tend to happen at about the same time that you begin to feel a bit low in your mood
   – Don't try to judge what you write at the time, just put it on paper and think it through later.
   – Some patients say that they don't have any **problem thoughts**; we usually find that this isn't the case. After a few days they get into the habit of looking and begin to notice them.
The message is: **please persevere!**

Look through the week and try to find out if the thoughts that have troubled you fall into the categories that we outlined above. The second help sheet will (we hope) make the task easier.

First help sheet

Day	Problem thoughts
Monday	
Tuesday	
Wednesday	
Thursday	
Friday	
Saturday	
Sunday	

Second help sheet

Put a tick next to the problem thought category that seems to fit the thoughts of the previous week:

1 Can you find any **absolutes** in the ways that you
   thought about some important problems? ☐ ☐
   ☐ ☐
   ☐ ☐
   ☐ ☐
   ☐ ☐

2 Were you **mind-reading**? ☐ ☐
   ☐ ☐
   ☐ ☐
   ☐ ☐
   ☐ ☐

3 **No win** situations
   Did you set yourself circumstances in which
   it wasn't possible to win? ☐ ☐
   ☐ ☐
   ☐ ☐
   ☐ ☐
   ☐ ☐

4 Did you tend to see yourself as the victim of
   your **diagnosis**? ☐ ☐
   ☐ ☐
   ☐ ☐
   ☐ ☐
   ☐ ☐

5 Did you **crystal ball gaze**? ☐ ☐
   ☐ ☐
   ☐ ☐
   ☐ ☐
   ☐ ☐

6 Did you tend to use the **mental magnifying glass**? ☐ ☐
   ☐ ☐
   ☐ ☐
   ☐ ☐
   ☐ ☐

7 Did you tend to play the **rejection record**? ☐ ☐
   ☐ ☐
   ☐ ☐
   ☐ ☐
   ☐ ☐

Third help sheet

First aid for problem thoughts

1 Try to notice how often the **problem thinking** happens each day

2 Try to notice at which times the **problem thinking** occurs each day

3 Try to notice if the **problem thinking** is associated with particular activities or events

4 Try to write down the **problem thoughts** and come back to them later, rather than trying to argue with yourself at the time

5 Try to pay particular attention to the words that you are using. See if it is possible to challenge them or put another point of view

6 Try to separate the contents of the **problem thoughts** into categories, then see if there is a particular sort of problem area which you could concentrate upon

7 Try to turn the **problem thought** from a definite statement of fact (that you may begin to believe) into a question. Sometimes the words that you use can stay the same. but the order can be changed. The following example will make this point a little clearer:
 – **I must** pretend that my tinnitus isn't ever a problem for me
 – **Must I** pretend that my tinnitus isn't ever a problem for me
 – **It is** always ...
 – **Is it** always ...
 – **People are** all the same
 – **Are people** all the same?

8 If you are upset by another person try to see if there could be another reason for them to act as they did. Is it true that the **only** reason that people do this is because they are thinking ...
 – If you feel upset because someone has seemed to be offhand for no reason, your first thought may be 'they know that I have tinnitus and can't be bothered to make allowance for this'. Try to look at the situation in an objective way. If you have already 'tried' and 'convicted' them of thoughtlessness it can be seen as good manners to be the defence solicitor as well. As we all know, everyone is presumed to be innocent initially, so evidence of their 'guilt' is required. The sort of questions which will tend to provide this information are:
 – Have they always acted in this way?
 – Do they have a reputation as an unkind person?
 – If another person was present ask for their opinion; did they think that you were treated badly?

– Think about the incident later. Are you **absolutely** sure that no other reason **whatever** could account for their behaviour? Ask for the opinion of others if you can't call alternatives easily to mind
– Could you have misunderstood the situation?
– If you put yourself into their place would you still think that they had **intended** to cause distress?

9 Above all, remember that although tinnitus is now a part of your life, other people may forget about it. We find that many patients are surprised that this happens. They have to remind others of their tinnitus, but when they do so, they are treated with kindness and consideration.

Fourth help sheet

This help sheet will concentrate of the ways that the categories of problem thoughts can be used to help improve your mood.

Select the category that seems to be the most important, then:
(a) Write the problem thoughts as they occur
(b) Challenge the thought
(c) Note any change in the thought
(d) Review your progress
(e) Start the process again from (a) but use the new knowledge to help.

1 Absolutes
– Absolutes include the following words
– Always
– Never
– Everyone
– Perfect
– Must

Challenge the words. Is it helpful to you to think in this way? Could you achieve your goals more easily if you took a more balanced view?

Are the difficulties which you have so vital to you or to the future of the world that no other choice exists?

2 Mind-reading
Look at a stranger: can you predict what they are going to say or do? We often can make an educated guess, but do we **know**? This may seem to be obvious, but why should you only be able to read minds when you are distressed by others?

3 No win
If you are setting yourself impossible targets, how can you blame yourself for failing to achieve them? If you have set yourself a challenge, ask yourself:

(a) Is it possible to achieve?
(b) Is it reasonable?
(c) Is it necessary?

4 Diagnosis

The diagnosis doesn't give an indication of how you will be affected by tinnitus. The diagnosis is not a personal description or a sentence of imprisonment. Put the tinnitus into its place as an unpleasant problem, but only one aspect of your life.

5 Crystal ball gazing

The future is unknown; this isn't an opinion but is widely held as a statement of fact. If we can only be 50% right when we toss a coin, is it reasonable to think that we can predict the course of a human life?

It may be possible that X will happen, it may be probable, it may be vital, but it **cannot be absolutely certain**. Therefore, why take the most pessimistic view as being a given fact? Try to look for a range of alternatives that are less distressing, but equally probable.

6 Mental magnifying glass

Challenge the thoughts by making sure that you have a 'reasonable person' in mind so that you can judge yourself and your problems. Think of your problems as being similar to a hot air balloon. The substance of both are very small but can grow rapidly, and can soon have control of us. They can sweep us away unless the hot air is controlled! See your problems as problems, not disasters.

7 Rejection record

Is the constant self-criticism helpful? If it doesn't seem to be helping you to achieve your goals what purpose does it serve?

Low mood makes self-criticism more likely than self-praise. However, if you look at how you are coping with your problems is it true to say that you are absolutely unable to find anything at all which is praiseworthy?

As we said earlier, the ability to challenge the problem thoughts isn't something which you are born with. Many people think that getting low mood is the equivalent of showing that you are weak or unable to cope. We hope that by now you will be able to find at least one good answer to this inaccurate and unhelpful view. The sort of person that you are obviously has an effect, but if that was the only reason that people became depressed, why have you been all right until now?

In addition, we can all imagine circumstances which even the most 'well balanced' individual would find distressing. For the vast majority of people in the vast majority of situations, challenging the thoughts will help! Therefore, try to use practise the techniques regularly in a variety of situations. We find that people make the most progress when they:

(a) use their skills at the times that they used to have problems

(b) practise regularly

(c) don't expect results straight away

(d) don't use the most difficult situations for practice.

Although it may seem to be an almost impossible to believe, tinnitus does not have to mean that you have constant low mood. With some help most people can overcome their (quite understandable) early distress. This assistance can, of course, come from your family and friends, your doctor or another clinician. However, the British Tinnitus Association (see 'Useful addresses' at the end of the book) can provide help and advice.

5 Overcoming insomnia

Chapter goals

By the end of this chapter we hope you:

1 Will be able to understand the link between your tinnitus and sleeping problems.
2 Will understand the contribution of your lifestyle to your sleeping problems.
3 Find ways of helping you to sleep as you would wish, using a number of different techniques.

Sleep is a much valued activity. A common morning greeting to our family and friends is 'Did you sleep well?' This is an indication of how important sleep is in our lives and reflects how troubled we become if our sleep is impaired for some reason. We are all keen to get a good night's sleep. Most people have some experience of sleeplessness and the debilitating effect it has such as tiredness, lethargy, a reduction in our ability to carry out our work and everyday tasks effectively, increased irritability and a lowering of our mood.

Occasional sleepless nights are commonplace and not too troublesome. However, for some people and often those suffering from tinnitus, occasional nights of sleep loss can develop into a picture of chronic and frequent insomnia. Many people seek to resolve this difficulty by taking sleeping tablets (hypnotics or tranquillisers). Whilst this may seem to be an effective remedy in the short term, in the longer term it can be fraught with problems (these are discussed later in this chapter in the section 'Treatment of insomnia using hypnotics and tranquillisers').

Almost everyone has an occasional night of disturbed sleep. These may typically occur when we have something important to do the next day, perhaps a job interview or a driving test. Sometimes sleep disturbance occurs during times of stress in our lives, when we have problems at work or problems in our families. Sometimes it may be due to having eaten too much at supper time or because of too much alcohol at a party. For others it will be related to their physical health, pain can impair sleep. Sometimes it is due to having to work shift patterns that are disruptive, for example, alternating between working day and night shifts. For many readers it is their tinnitus sounds that seem to prevent them getting off to sleep. Sometimes it is very difficult to relate our poor sleep to any specific current problems or events. For some of us our insomnia may last for a few nights but for others it may persist for many years.

Insomnia, like tinnitus, is not a disease but a symptom. It is a subjective complaint for which there is no agreed definition. This is because individuals differ widely in the amount of sleep required to ensure they feel rested. Each of us has a kind of personal optimum or ideal, but for some it might be as little as only 3 hours a night whilst others may require as much as 10 hours of uninterrupted sleep to feel refreshed. We know that the often quoted 8 hours a night is only a guide. Many of us need much more, others much less. In addition to this difference between people, we do not have a 'fixed for ever requirement'.

Categories of insomnia

Doctors recognise three main kinds of sleep problems. The most common sleep disorder is of difficulty getting off to sleep. It has been estimated that three quarters of people seeking help with sleep problems fall into this category, which is sometimes called 'sleep onset insomnia'. Although it may take people with this problem several hours to get off to sleep, once they are asleep they tend to sleep without further interruption.

A second and common form of sleep disturbance 'intermittent insomnia', a problem in which the maintenance of sleep is disrupted. Individuals with this problem may get off to sleep quite satisfactorily but may wake in the middle of the night and have considerable difficulty getting off to sleep again or may awaken frequently throughout the night impairing the quality of their sleep.

A third type is 'early morning awakening', when the individual awakens several hours before their intended or desired time with an inability to get back off to sleep. This latter kind of problem is usually seen in people with problems of often quite severe depression.

For many people, poor sleep might consist of any or all of these three kinds of sleep problems or may simply be experienced as sleep of poor quality, that feels too light, or in which the person has felt themselves to be restless.

Size of the problem

Surveys have shown that only 5% of the adult population claimed never to have sleeping difficulties. 95% of us have problems sleeping some of the time, and one in five regarded their sleeping problem as serious. In a large survey carried out in the USA, almost a third of adults questioned said they had a current problem of insomnia. A survey of 4000 physicians in America found that 18% of their patients complained of insomnia. Insomnia seems to be more frequently reported by females (perhaps twice as frequently as males), and by thinner people, and there is a considerable body of reports to show that complaints of insomnia increase with age.

Surprisingly, there is little information available about the extent of sleep problems in people who suffer from tinnitus.

Tinnitus and insomnia

There are two main factors that cause sleep problems in tinnitus sufferers. The major factor is simply that the tinnitus noises keep people awake. A less important cause is concerned with the relatively high incidence of tinnitus in older people and the relationship, as mentioned above, between older age and more frequent complaints of insomnia (older people with tinnitus have the cards stacked against them!).

For tinnitus sufferers, going to sleep can the a major problem. As you turn off the light, close your eyes and lay your head on the pillow, you may become increasingly aware of the disruptive effects of your tinnitus noises. By closing your eyes you are substantially reducing the stimulation to your brain (because you have 'switched off' all the stimuli that come through your eyes). As mentioned earlier your tinnitus noises are competing for your attention. By switching off the light and closing your eyes you are giving a big advantage to the noises competing for your brain's attention.

Secondly, it is very likely that you choose to sleep in a room that is relatively quiet and again, by reducing the sensory input to your brain (this time via your ears and auditory channels), you are handing over the advantage to your tinnitus noises.

A third disadvantage arises from the tinnitus noises themselves. The noises, particularly when heard against a background of relative peace and quiet in a darkened room, may be perceived as quite unpleasant and aversive. The effects of this may be to make you tense, to increase your state of physical and mental arousal. These states are incompatible with sleep and you are sentenced to a period or night of sleeplessness.

A fourth source of interference with sleep may arise from your worry and anxiety about not getting to sleep. As you were unable to sleep last night and have something important to do tomorrow (such as getting to work on time) you may become tense and anxious at the prospect of not sleeping or having insufficient sleep to let you cope well the next day. As mentioned in the paragraph above, these are ideal conditions for keeping you wide awake! This concern may be magnified if you begin to worry about keeping your partner awake by your restlessness as you seek a comfortable sleeping position. Sleep failure breeds sleep failure because the mere anticipation of failing to get off to sleep quickly may signal to you that you are about to fail again.

Consequences of insomnia

Occasional sleep-disturbed nights are generally of little consequence. Such occurrences may cause minor annoyance but our bodies and minds return to their normal state within days at most. However, with persistent insomnia the situation can be quite different.

There is plenty of evidence to show that our ability to carry out our normal daily activities of work, engage in social activities, feel mentally and physically well, may he seriously impaired. It is difficult to think of any of our activities and feelings that are not seriously compromised by chronic insomnia. One of the prominent symptoms of chronic sleep deprivation is a feeling of tiredness during the day, particularly when engaging in sedentary activities. Sometimes this state is accompanied by feelings of tension, irritability, short temper and low mood. Your normal zest for living and ability to enjoy life may disappear. Adverse and negative feelings may themselves begin to interfere and disrupt relationships at home and at work. There is some evidence to demonstrate that persons with insomnia are more likely to complain of general health problems.

For tinnitus sufferers insomnia may present even more of a problem because many will look forward to sleep as a time when they will not have to put up with unpleasant intrusive noises in their ear. Sleep for many is their only true escape from the noises. Insomnia in tinnitus sufferers leads to a cycle of problems in that the negative physical and mental states induced by chronic insomnia make the ability to tolerate and cope with tinnitus noises much more difficult. As mentioned earlier, any adverse physical or emotional state makes the experience of tinnitus a substantially greater problem.

Treatment of insomnia using hypnotics and tranquillisers

The most common method for treating insomnia with medication is the use of sleep-inducing drugs, called hypnotics and tranquillisers. In a British survey, 23% of adults surveyed had taken either tranquillisers or hypnotics at some time and of these, 35% had taken them for more than four months. However over recent years the number of prescriptions for such drugs has declined.

At first glance, the use of hypnotics and tranquillisers to aid sleep seems to be a reasonable solution to the problem. The medication is relatively inexpensive, and is easy to take with few side effects. However the first problem that users encounter is that although the drugs tend to be good at getting them off to sleep, and sometimes prolonging sleep duration if the appropriate dosage is given, they quickly cease to be as effective. In other words, after only a few weeks of starting to take them your body will start to become used to them and higher dosages will be required to achieve the same effect that you initially experienced. Some hypnotics (the short–acting ones) work by helping you to sleep, but do not keep you asleep (as the longer–acting ones do). The shorter–acting ones are preferable because tolerance to them seems to develop more slowly and they are regarded as safer. A second problem is of possible dependence, resulting in withdrawal symptoms on stopping. The withdrawal symptoms may include restlessness and insomnia!

Hypnotics are generally recommended for only short term treatment of sleep disturbance, for example, at times of personal crises. They are also useful for chronically sleep impaired individuals, to provide a respite of sleep, although it is important to resist the urge to increase the dosage.

Some people turn to alcohol as an aid to sleep. Alcohol acts on the central nervous system as a depressant and,in effect, it acts as an anaesthetic. This drug is not to be recommended for many of the reasons given for not using hypnotics and tranquillisers. The evidence shows that whilst small amounts of alcohol may help relax a tense person and thus aid sleep, any quantity of alcohol will actually disrupt the quality of sleep. Alcohol–induced sleep tends to be characterised by frequent awakenings and disturbed dreams, resulting in sleep that is not particularly restful. It is a dangerous drug, particularly when taken with hypnotics and tranquillisers.

Perhaps the most important disadvantage of hypnotics and tranquillisers is that they take away your own natural ability to sleep. They prevent you from developing or renewing your own personal ability to manage sleep naturally. They eradicate your feelings of personal control as you depend on external sources (medication) to facilitate sleep.

The remaining sections in this chapter are concerned with helping you find alternative methods of overcoming insomnia.

Overcoming insomnia

This section will be concerned with establishing guidelines to ensure you develop a satisfactory sleeping pattern. Some of the guidelines are concerned with eliminating actions which make it difficult for you to get off to sleep, but most will be about things you can do to positively encourage sleeping success.

Before we embark on the suggestions that we recommend that you adopt to overcome insomnia, it is important to establish some means of assessing, or measuring your current sleep problem. Before trying any of the guidelines, keep a record of your sleep for two weeks first using the sleep diary (Table 5.1). Keep a record of your answers to these questions using the form in Table 5.2.

Table 5.1 Daily sleep diary

1 What time did you go to bed last night? _____

2 How long did it take you to fall asleep last night? _____

3 How many times did you awaken during the night? _____

4 How long were you awake for on each occasion? _____

_____   _____

5 How long did you sleep for, altogether last night? _____

6 How noisy were your tinnitus sounds when you went to bed last night?

0	1	2	3	4	5
Not noisy					As noisy as they have ever been

7 How relaxed were you when you went to bed last night?

0	1	2	3	4	5
Very tense					Very relaxed

8 How rested do you feel this morning?

0	1	2	3	4	5
Very rested					Poorly rested

9 Rate the quality of last night's sleep

0	1	2	3	4	5
Very poor					Excellent

10 Did you take any sleeping tablets last night? yes/no

If yes, what were they? _____

Sleep and high levels of stimulation and tension are incompatible. Smoking, either prior to going to bed or during periods when you might awaken in the night is not to be recommended. Nicotine, from cigarettes, is a central nervous system stimulant. It acts by alerting our brain; this is not what we want to do if we wish to fall asleep! The evidence is that in a group of chronic insomniacs, those who smoke will on average take much longer to get off to sleep than non-smokers. When smokers refrain from smoking the time it takes for them to get off to sleep falls. The sleep of smokers may also be interfered with by coughing which may awaken them (or their partners).

Table 5.2 Sleep diary record

Question number	Days													
	1	2	3	4	5	6	7	8	9	10	11	12	13	14
1														
2														
3														
4														
5														
6														
7														
8														
9														
10														

Suggestion 1. If you do smoke, try not to smoke within an hour or two of your bedtime

Another central nervous system stimulant is caffeine which is present in coffee, cola drinks and to a lesser extent in tea. Although individuals vary in their sensitivity to caffeine, the effects of taking it will last for several hours with the most noticeable effect occurring an hour after drinking it. Stimulants are also to be found in a range of medications including some cold remedies, decongestants, and drugs to treat migraine and asthma, steroids and bronchodilators.

Suggestion 2. Try to eliminate unnecessary stimulants, particularly caffeine, for several hours before bedtime

For the reasons given earlier in this chapter it is important not to regularly use alcohol as a means of getting to sleep.

Suggestion 3 Do not use alcohol to aid sleep

Some people, on retiring to bed, begin to think about the things they did during the day, or begin to worry about particular problems they might have, including worrying about whatever might be coming along the next day. This kind of activity, if it excites or worries you, is certainly not to be recommended, simply because it alerts you. As mentioned earlier, this is incompatible with getting to sleep. Although we might debate about whether worrying is an unavoidable state, we believe that worrying, can be deferred to a better time. Worrying shouldn't be a thing you do in bed!

Spending your time in pleasurable anticipation of forthcoming events, too, might be unhelpful. Try to defer your worrying by deciding to do it next day. Try to relax (using the techniques in Chapter 4) and neutralise any tension you have. If you use a relaxation tape as a means of becoming relaxed, it is worthwhile playing your tape as you retire to bed, as this will relax your muscles and help you empty your mind of worrying thoughts.

Suggestion 4. Bedtime is not a time for worrying, try to relax

The following section is a quick quiz to see whether you have understood and learned some basic information about caffeine and sensible things to do to aid sleep. The answers are given at the end of the chapter.

Please indicate which of the following list contain caffeine, by writing **YES** next to it:

Tea	Beer
Aspirin	Chocolate cake
Lemonade	Sleeping pills
Coffee	Wine

The 'good sleep' checklist

Please indicate which of the following items in the list help you to get to sleep by writing yes next to it:

1 Having a nap in the daytime
2 Having a cup of tea or coffee before going to bed
3 Going to bed at the same time each night
4 Going to bed hungry
5 Setting aside time to relax before going to bed
6 Going to bed thirsty
7 Drinking more than three glasses of wine or beer in the evening
8 Smoking more than 20 cigarettes a day
9 Thinking about problems when trying to sleep

So far in this section we have not made any reference to the particular problems faced by tinnitus sufferers. As mentioned earlier, the reasons why tinnitus sufferers have particular problems is that on retiring to bed they close their eyes (thus shutting out all visual stimulation) in a room that is quiet and as they put their heads on the pillow their tinnitus noises seem to be magnified.

Paradoxically perhaps, many tinnitus sufferers have been able to overcome this problem by creating additional noise to 'mask' or cover their tinnitus noise. Some sufferers provide this sound by introducing a loudly ticking clock into their bedrooms, others have recommended playing a radio and some prefer to use the masker they wear during the day. It is possible to buy little gadgets that produce gentle hissing sounds, rather like the sounds of the sea breaking on the shore. This approach requires an element of trial and error, trying out various sound sources to mask your own individual tinnitus noises.

Suggestion 5. Create sounds in your bedroom to 'mask' your tinnitus noises

Chronic sleep problems do not develop overnight and will not disappear very quickly either. It is important to set yourself a realistic series of goals or targets. Your first goal should be to ensure that you are following each of the five rules mentioned above. Once these are established 'habits' we would like you to try to adopt the following new rules for sleeping. They are based on a great deal of research an evaluation on persons with chronic sleep problems, although it is true that sleep research seems to have ignored the problems of tinnitus sufferers.

Many of us will have used a variety of 'tricks' to aid sleep, such as going out for a walk, having a warm bath, or taking a hot milk drink immediately prior to going to bed. Some people, on retiring to bed, watch TV, smoke, eat food, read books and magazines. Some of these activities can be useful but are often variable in their usefulness. For example, reading may sometimes make us feel tired; alternatively it might stimulate us.

We strongly recommend that if you have a permanent problem of difficulty getting to sleep, that you try the following programme. It can be a tough programme to follow but will pay dividends once you ensure you follow all the rules:

Self control procedures for overcoming insomnia

1 Go to your bedroom to sleep **only** when you feel sleepy. Stick to this even if it means your going to bed much later than your 'normal' time.

2 Set your alarm for the same time each morning, irrespective of how much (or how little) sleep you have had the previous night or during the day.

3 When you go to bed you should try to relax as much as you can. **Do not** under any circumstances, read, watch TV, listen to the radio, smoke, chat, drink or eat in bed. Your bed is only for sleeping in!

4 If you are not asleep within about twenty minutes of going to bed, get up and go into another room.

5 When in another room you should do something relaxing such as reading or listening to music. Do not do anything active or energetic. Return to your bedroom **only** if you feel sleepy.

6 If on returning to bed you do not fall asleep within twenty minutes, repeat step 4.

7 Do not sleep during the day.

Some of these rules require explanation, and perhaps justification. It is important to go to your bedroom only when you feel sleepy because if you go before this you are likely to lie in bed awake, wishing you were asleep. It may be that this means going to bed considerably later than your normal time and you will worry that, as you have to get up at a fixed time to get to work, you will not have enough sleep. This programme has short term 'costs' of perhaps sleep deprivation (which you already have), but the benefits will substantially outweigh these costs.

It is very important that you arise at a fixed time every day (including weekends and holidays), otherwise you will find that you simply move your sleep problem to a different time of the day. If you have had very little sleep one night because you went to bed late but still get up at a fixed time, you will feel sleep–

deprived and tired. Consequently, you will be much more likely to sleep well the next night. Over a number of nights, perhaps two or three weeks, you will begin to establish a regular sleep cycle.

The third rule is concerned with treating your bedroom as somewhere exclusively reserved for sleeping, thus creating an association between being in bed and sleeping (rather than lying in bed wide awake). It is important not to lie in bed beyond the initial twenty minutes because you are likely to start becoming anxious about not falling asleep which, as mentioned earlier in this chapter, will alert you and prevent you falling asleep. Go into another room, but don't do anything that is likely to make you more alert. Only return when you feel sleepy (whatever the time), as you won't sleep until you are sleepy. On returning to bed there is no point lying there beyond a further twenty minutes; you know why. Don't sleep during the day as you will defeat and undermine the efforts you have made in following the programme. If you find yourself about to have a nap on the couch, get up and take some fresh air.

We can't overstate the importance of keeping a regular sleep diary. If you maintain a diary from before embarking on the programme and for several weeks afterwards you will begin to see a number of changes which hopefully will consist of a reduction in the time it takes for you to get off to sleep, and in the number of times you awaken in the night. Your amount of sleep will increase, your tinnitus will become less troublesome, and you will begin to generate a sleeping pattern that leaves you feeling much more rested.

We are confident that you will substantially overcome your sleep problem by following the rules and advice given in this chapter. You need to keep trying don't give up!

Earlier in this chapter we asked you to keep a daily sleep diary for two weeks before embarking on the programme outlined above. About four weeks after you have tried to put the advice into practice, reassess your sleep problem by completing the diary in Table 5.3 and compare your answers with your previous answers. We confidently expect to see some marked improvement. Reassess again in three months time and again compare. If you have followed the advice faithfully but have not improved significantly, it may be worthwhile asking your family doctor to refer you for professional help from your local clinical psychology department.

Table 5.3 Daily sleep diary

---

1 What time did you go to bed last night? _____

2 How long did it take you to fall asleep last night? _____

3 How many times did you awaken during the night? _____

4 How long were you awake for on each occasion? _____

_____   _____   _____

5 How long did you sleep for, altogether, last night? _____

6 How noisy were your tinnitus sounds when you went to bed last night?

0	1	2	3	4	5
Not noisy					As noisy as they have ever been

7 How relaxed were you when you went to bed last night?

0	1	2	3	4	5
Very tense					Very relaxed

8 How rested do you feel this morning?

0	1	2	3	4	5
Very rested					Poorly rested

9 Rate the quality of last night's sleep

0	1	2	3	4	5
Very poor					Excellent

10 Did you take any sleeping tablets last night? yes/no

If yes, what were they? _____

We are confident that you will substantially overcome your sleep problem by following, the rules and advice given in this chapter. You need to keep trying; don't give up!

Answers to quiz

Caffeine knowledge
The answers are given in brackets

Tea [yes]	Beer [no]
Aspirin [no]	Chocolate cake [yes]
Lemonade [no]	Sleeping pills [no]
Coffee [yes]	Wine [no]

The 'good sleep' checklist
The answers are given in brackets

1 Having a nap in the daytime [no]
2 Having a cup of tea or coffee before going to bed [no]
3 Going to bed at the same time each night [yes]
4 Going to bed hungry [no]
5 Setting aside time to relax before going to bed [yes]
6 Going to bed thirsty [no]
7 Drinking more than three glasses of wine or beer in the evening [no]
8 Smoking more than 20 cigarettes a day [no]
9 Thinking about problems when trying to sleep [no]

6 Changing environments

Chapter goals

By the end of this chapter we hope that you:

1 Understand the methods that you can use to alter your environment.
2 Recognise the link between your environment and the degree of distress which tinnitus causes.
3 Act to reduce your difficulties, using the strategies outlined in the chapter.

This chapter is concerned with methods of changing your environment so that some of the problems caused by your tinnitus can be effectively overcome.

Basically there are only four strategies for dealing with this problem:

1 *Make changes to your social environment.* Briefly, this may involve informing family and friends of some of the difficulties tinnitus gives you and asking for their help and understanding. You may ask them to change their behaviour in some way and you may wish to consider whether you ought to try to see things in a different way.

2 *Use distraction techniques.* You will know already that your tinnitus is either absent or much less of a problem if you are absorbed in something that is interesting. You will have discovered that if you are distracted by something that requires your attention you are less troubled by tinnitus noises.

3 *Mask your tinnitus sounds.* External sounds which mask or cover up your noises can bring relief. This can be achieved in many cases by either changing your environment to one in which there is much background noise, for example by having the radio on, or by wearing a masker.

4 *Avoid difficult situations or leave when you can't cope.* Of the four strategies listed, unfortunately this may be the one with which you are most familiar. How often have you decided not to go somewhere or do something for fear of it either being too

difficult to tolerate with having tinnitus or too risky in terms of making your tinnitus worse? Similarly, how many times have you had to leave a situation because you felt you couldn't cope?

Most people would agree that the first three methods are better than the fourth. The first three are concerned with coping with or overcoming the problems caused by tinnitus, whilst the fourth is an indication of not coping. That is not to say, however, that there are not times when it is perfectly sensible and wise to avoid some situations (we all do this, don't we?) and others when leaving is better than staying. The key point is the reasons or excuses we allow ourselves to make for avoiding or escaping.

In this chapter we will investigate, in some detail, all four methods or strategies for overcoming the problems caused by tinnitus noises.

1 Make changes to your social environment

Your tinnitus noises affect not only you but also, indirectly, family members and friends. When they first learn of your tinnitus problem they will be curious about it and undoubtedly sympathetic. For a while they may be happy for you to tell them how awful it can be and how much of a nuisance the noises are in interfering with your ability to tolerate some situations. They will, for a time, make conscious efforts to try to ensure that your needs are considered. After a while, however, this goodwill will become less obvious. It may seem that family and friends have forgotten your plight or act as if your problem, like their apparent concern, has ebbed away.

We have returned to the theme that one of the problems for someone with tinnitus is that their difficulty is not visible.

One patient we know who was hard of hearing always wore his hearing aid on the outside of his clothes in public situations, but never switched it on. He discovered that people, on noticing his hearing aid, either shouted to make him hear or else took the trouble to articulate their words more carefully.

For the tinnitus sufferer, such subtle indicators of a possible 'handicap' are not available. How do you make others aware of your difficulties? One patient always wore cotton wool in both of her ears in order to signal the message that those was something wrong with her ears, if not specifically that she had tinnitus. She felt that this increased the likelihood that others would be sympathetic in some way.

As mentioned earlier in this book, it is possible to obtain an audiotape of simulated tinnitus noises which you can play to family and friends. This will give them some indication of the noises that you may be tormented by, but unfortunately gives them little prospect about how they themselves would cope if they had tinnitus. How could they know what it is really like to have tinnitus? How can they estimate their own ability to tolerate and overcome tinnitus? We have worked for some years with a wide variety of patients with conditions such as anxiety, depression, alcoholism, obesity, physical handicaps, and some, who may have been sexually abused or have a terminal cancer. Whilst we can try to empathise with them, we have not experienced some of their symptoms and will always have some difficulty in knowing what it is really like, for example to have tinnitus.

On the other hand, sometimes your sympathetic family and friends remind you that you have tinnitus and it is this focussing on tinnitus noises that you wish to avoid. The more often you remind others of your tinnitus the more likely they are to raise this with you an unhelpful circle to be avoided.

The most crucial aspect to consider is whether your social life has been affected by your having tinnitus. Ask yourself these questions:

Am I doing less than I used to because I have tinnitus ?

What reasons do I have for not doing as much as I used to ?

This latter question requires some attention. Is it really only tinnitus that has stopped you doing some things? Is it the tinnitus itself or some consequence of it? For example, have you lost some of your confidence to do some things? Are you frightened that some situations (such as noisy places) will make your tinnitus worse? Have you lost interest in such things? Do you ever use your tinnitus as an excuse to your family and friends (and yourself) for avoiding situations or leaving before the end? This last question may be particularly difficult for you to answer.

Cancelling an occasional social event or turning, down an invitation now and again is probably reasonable and acceptable to others, but avoiding these frequently will inevitably lead to either a reduction in invitations or, worse still, a belief you might develop of not wanting to participate in social activities. You might actually convince yourself that you prefer to do nothing!

However, this may develop into feelings of isolation, and ultimately hopelessness and emptiness.

One way of addressing these questions, to discover whether it is really your tinnitus that is stopping you, is to monitor your tinnitus over a period of time. For one month, accept all invitations and if these are few try to establish opportunities for socialising. Keep a daily record of how you coped with each situation in terms of whether it was pleasurable, how severe your tinnitus was, and the ways in which your tinnitus interfered with your ability to socialise and enjoy yourself.

Consider what you can learn from your records. You are likely to discover that it is not necessarily the people or situations that are problematic, but the severity of your tinnitus on that occasion. In other words, your tinnitus noises and interference level will vary both within and between situations. On one occasion you will be unaware or barely aware of the noises, but in the same situation on another occasion there may be problems. Are there things you can do within situations to cope more effectively? Later in this chapter we shall look at distraction or absorption techniques. We will be looking at ways to distract you from the tinnitus noises and help you become more absorbed in what is going on.

If you can gain some measure of control over your tinnitus noises, what thing would you like to do again and what new things would you like to tackle?

Another aspect is to stop regarding yourself as a tinnitus sufferer. In many places throughout the book we have referred to you as a tinnitus sufferer. We feel this is justified because those who don't regard themselves as sufferers are less likely to read the book. However, **we want you to stop regarding yourself as a tinnitus sufferer**. By following the advice and guidance contained in the book, we confidently expect that the suffering caused by having tinnitus will be minimised.

Whilst you are still absorbing these ideas, try to stop being a tinnitus sufferer for the next few minutes or for the rest of the day. This means doing all the things you would do if you didn't have tinnitus and **stop talking about it**! The following section describes how this may be achieved.

2 Use distraction techniques

It is necessary to know something about what psychologists refer to as 'attention'. Our brains are like computers in that they receive information, process it, and display part of this on the visual display unit or TV screen, and may put some into their memory stores. Our brains constantly receive input from our senses. Simultaneously, our brains are receiving visual input from our eyes, auditory input from our ears, perhaps olfactory or smell input from our noses, maybe taste input from our tongues, and a whole host of information from our bodies in terms of touch and the position of various parts of our bodies in space (our brains know, for example, the position of our hands).

This is a mass of sensory input but of course our conscious selves are not aware of much of the input until we pay attention to it. You were probably not paying attention to the pressure of your buttocks on the chair you are sitting on until you read this sentence. You may be ignoring the ticking of that clock or even the noises of your tinnitus (which suggests you are paying close attention to what you're reading)

You are unable to experience all the information you are capable of sensing at any point in time. You can only attend to a limited amount. What is it that determines which sensory input is attended to? If the telephone starts to ring, if a car backfires outside on the road, or if you can smell toast burning, you will find that your attention switches to these. These are novel sensory input in that they are stimuli which stand out from the background stimuli or 'noise' that you are in contact with. Our attention automatically switches to pay attention to these stimuli which may momentarily distract us from what we are doing.

Some very complex activities may require very little conscious attention. If you are a car driver you will no doubt recall how very complex the act of simultaneously pressing your left foot on the clutch, moving the gear stick with your left hand and looking to see around the corner which you are just approaching, never mind the requirement to be prepared for a child stepping off the pavement, or listening to the car radio. Eventually, we are able to drive our car without really having to think very hard. Our attention channel is by no means full and we have some spare capacity to concentrate on something else. However, when driving, our attention can very rapidly switch to some stimulus such as the sight and sounds of a police car and often our first reaction is to slow down and look at the car's speedometer.

Nature has equipped us to ignore much of the stimuli or sensory material that comes our way. We do not listen to our own breathing (unless of course there is a change in rate or if we have some kind of illness), and don't spend conscious effort listening, to the clock ticking away on our mantelpiece. We have got into the habit of ignoring such noises.

Tinnitus noises too, may become ignored with time. Psychologists have referred to this ignoring by habit mechanism as 'habituation'. Unfortunately, many people with tinnitus never establish habituation and continue to pay some attention to their tinnitus sounds. Part of the reason for habituation failure is the negative or emotional flavour of the noises. We are preprogrammed to pay attention to material which has an emotional component (hence the use of emotional material in advertising). A series of experiments showed that if you present people with long lists of words they are much more likely to remember those with some kind of emotional flavour.

Let's try this out. Get a piece of paper and pen. Below is a list of 40 words. Read them out aloud, count up to 30, turn the book over and write down as many of the words as you can.

HOUSE	CYCLE	VAGINA	PAPER	TELEVISION
BREAST	PENIS	PENCIL	TAMPAX	TREE
ELEPHANT	CLITORIS	SCOOTER	BOOK	COMPASS
ORGASM	CLOWN	TINNITUS	TELEPHONE	PICTURE
ARM	BOAT	SCROTUM	FOLDER	CLOCK	HORSE
BUTTOCKS	ARMCHAIR	COCK	TABLE	CARPET
CUP	INTERCOURSE	RADIO	SATCHEL	MOUSE
COMB	DESK	STAR	SEX

How many words were you able to recall? There were 12 emotionally loaded words (11 with sexual connotations and the word tinnitus) and 28 emotionally neutral (we hope) words. That is, 30% of the words had an emotional flavour. If you count how many words you correctly recalled, have you discovered that more than 30% were from the emotionally loaded list of words?

As another example of our pre-programming to pay attention

to certain stimuli, consider the mother of a young baby who seems to develop acute hearing for detecting that her baby is crying (where the baby's father seems not to have heard).

In many ways, tinnitus might be viewed as a disorder of attention. Tinnitus sounds have little apparent usefulness to us. We ought to stop attending to tinnitus noises, as we stop attending to the ticking of clocks.

When your tinnitus first appeared it is likely that much of your waking time was spent paying attention to the noises and you were well aware of how much it was interfering with your everyday activities. However you might accept that the tinnitus sounds were not being attended to all of the time in those early days. You had to divert your attention away from the sounds to carry out activities such as thinking which, at least momentarily, will have taken your full attention or concentration.

Distraction is a very simple technique. It is not a cure for tinnitus, but simply a technique which you can use in many situations in which tinnitus noises interfere. Distraction involves switching your attention from the tinnitus noise and your consequent distress to absolutely anything else which requires full attention or concentration. By paying attention to a distractor there will not be room in your attention 'channel' to allow tinnitus noises in.

If you are engaged in a conversation within a small group and your noises interfere, try to concentrate on what is being said have a close look at the person who is speaking. Do their gestures and body posture fit in with the words they are using? By the time you have addressed these two things (concentrating on what is being said and their gestures and body posture) your tinnitus noises will have been pushed out.

Of course, in some situations you are alone and required to pay attention to other stimuli. If none are apparent to you, you can try to think! Thinking is a powerful distracter. If you have nothing to think about, try multiplying some numbers together in your head or see if you can make your shoulders relaxed.

Keeping 'busy' is not usually the answer. There are so many things we do that we do without having to think or pay much attention. Housework (like driving mentioned above) is one of these activities. It is not related to the complexity of the task as much as the ongoing attention required to do it. You can dust very precious porcelain figures with great care but your mind can be elsewhere. If your mind is capable of being 'elsewhere' it is equally capable of paying attention to tinnitus noises!

If you are capable of switching your attention away from the tinnitus noises you are, in effect, capable of switching them off.

As you will see in Chapter 7, the use of visual imagery to generate pleasant images can be enormously useful. If you are capable of switching your attention away from the tinnitus noises you are, in effect, capable of switching them off!

3 Mask your tinnitus sounds

You may well have discovered that your tinnitus noises are less intense, intrusive and troublesome if you are in a noisy environment. As discussed in the previous chapter on insomnia, your perception of tinnitus noises in very quiet rooms, such as your bedroom at night, is of increased volume. Noisy environments tend to reduce the apparent loudness and nuisance value of tinnitus noises because they cover them up. This strategy works because generally tinnitus noises are quieter than everyday sounds outside of your head. These louder sounds effectively erase the tinnitus noises inside your head.

Many of our patients obtain relief by either seeking out noisy environments or by creating their own e.g. by playing their radio as background noise. This approach is a matter of 'hit and miss' and you might like to try it for yourself. Several of our patients have found benefit from using portable cassette players and have experimented with various kinds of music. Some claim that the works of Mozart are best, but this may reflect their musical preference rather than be an indication of the physical qualities of the masking sounds produced.

A more scientific and usually more accurate and satisfactory way to mask tinnitus noises is to have a tinnitus masker fitted.

Types of maskers. Tinnitus maskers became available nearly fifteen years ago. There are five types available currently:

(a) Behind the ear – this device looks like a behind-the-ear hearing aid. The noise generated is a kind of swishing sound which can be adjusted for volume. The various models vary in the pitch of sound generated and in volume.

(b) In the ear – this device is an ear canal masker which is fitted to a standard ear mould. It is readily fitted and is comfortable to wear all day (and night too).

(c) Dual device – This is a combined hearing aid and masker aimed at people with tinnitus with appreciable hearing loss. Some of our patients have found them to be a little tricky to use as it is essential to set the volume control on the hearing aid firstly, and then the masker. As with all maskers, the ideal is to use the lowest possible volume setting that effectively masks out the tinnitus noises.

(d) Adjustable maskers – these are programmable devices that are worn on the body. Their essential difference is that they can be adjusted to produce a range of sounds that more closely match the sounds produced by the assessment equipment available to audiological technicians and ENT specialists in their clinic.

(e) Other devices – these are not worn on the body but are simply sound generators that you might wish to use at home. The commonest form is a white noise generator for use as an aid to sleep. It is a small box that can produce noises which sound like the sea, the waves, the wind (slushing and swishing sounds).

How do maskers work?

There are several possible explanations why maskers might provide relief. Unlike the majority of tinnitus noises, the sounds generated by maskers are constant and consequently easier to habituate to. In other words, it is easier to ignore noises which are meaningless and lack novel qualities. Earlier in this chapter we discussed how our brains selectively attend to various stimuli and how we ignore stimuli such as sounds if they lack novel qualities, have no meaning or are repeated constantly.

Another explanation is that the masker sounds, although slightly louder than your tinnitus noise, are a more acceptable sound. In Chapter 7 we shall look at imagery. Essentially, we believe that tinnitus noises which are distressing understandably become regarded by the sufferer in a very negative way, and their presence can set up an emotional response. Masker sounds, on the other hand, are likely to regarded in a neutral way, no anxiety or lowering in mood is produced and they become accepted with their perhaps soothing tranquillising effect.

Some people have suggested that maskers work and are acceptable because the wearer is able to establish personal control over the sounds in that they can adjust the volume, turn it off, etc. There are many situations in which we feel more contented if we feel we have a good deal of control or influence over things.

An interesting observation in a small minority of patients is that when the masker is switched off the relief from tinnitus continues! Complete absence of tinnitus noises in this situation are rare, but many users derive partial and temporary relief. This process has been called reciprocal inhibition.In some patients the effects of reciprocal inhibition are so great that the patients can gain good relief by using their masker for only a couple of hours a day, perhaps for an hour on waking, and similarly for the hour prior to sleep. Unfortunately, the reciprocal inhibition effect is not readily predicted. The masker user should experiment with various masking sounds and pitches to see whether they can generate this effect. It seems that the best way to see whether you can get the reciprocal inhibition effect is to increase the volume of your masker above the minimal level you use for masking for short period. **Some caution is required.** It is important not to play your masker on full volume without discussing this with your audiological technician or ENT specialist as some maskers generate sound at levels which may be potentially damaging (i.e. above 85 decibels).

We know of no evidence that maskers are in any way unsafe but it is important to bear in mind, as noted above, that the maximum volume output of some devices may be higher than 85 decibels. There is always the danger that for some individuals the masker will be only partially effective at low volumes. The temptation is to try greater and greater volumes to obtain relief. If you have any doubts or concerns about the safety (or potential benefits) of maskers, please be sure to discuss this with your audiological technician or ENT specialist. You may have to settle for partial masking success which is certainly better than nothing.

Do maskers work?

This is a very simple and straightforward question. The answer, however, is not so simple and straightforward. There is no doubt that if a comprehensive service is provided to the potential wearer the chances of benefits are substantially increased. The masker needs to be fitted with care, information should be provided about the best ways to use the device, and there need to be opportunities for follow-up visits to discuss problems encountered,

Surveys have suggested that many patients are unwilling to try them, and many give up using them after only a short time. Many do not use them often enough in any period to be able to know whether they will be of benefit. We know, however, of patients who are given maskers and when they return to the audiology clinic for check-ups they fail to inform staff that they have not been using their masker. Some even report that the masker is helping when it is not. Occasionally, some patients take the view that they don't like to disappoint the clinic staff and they fail to tell them of the failure of the masker. Clinic staff depend on your honest feedback on whatever help is tried. If it isn't working and you have done what you agreed to do, please say so!

Surveys suggest that approximately half of sufferers will successfully mask their tinnitus noises. This result seems pretty impressive. However, in one study subjects were asked to try a device that supposedly delivered a small electrical current to the ear and this was found to be as beneficial as using a masker. We take a pragmatic view. As maskers help a substantial proportion of patients we believe they are worth providing.

One of the interesting spin-offs from masker use is the benefits obtained by some people who have become frightened of loud noises. A small proportion of our patients have become apprehensive about loud noises for a variety of reasons. For some it is almost like a phobia, a phonophobia, which is characterised by avoiding noisy places or having to leave prematurely. Simply the thought of entering noisy environments can provoke anxiety.

Psychologists usually treat people with phobias by gradually exposing them to their feared situation. Imagine someone who is frightened of spiders. They may not be able to tolerate even looking at pictures of spiders without feelings of anxiety and revulsion. The psychologist would first show them a series of spiders, gradually introducing examples of more and more frightening ones. After a while the patient can tolerate this perfectly readily. The next steps may be to show them a small dead spider sealed in a glass jar. The next step may be to show them a live spider, again quite small, in a sealed jar. At first, they may be reluctant to hold the jar, even though they know logically that the spider will not be able to get out and run on their hand. Gradually, they might be introduced to larger spiders or they might handle a glass jar without a top with a small spider inside. Eventually they will be able to tolerate having a large house spider on the floor by their feet and will be able to catch it in a jar.

The same kind of treatment programme can be used with people frightened of noise. Later in this chapter we shall describe how to overcome this fear in social situations. For masker wearers the spin-off mentioned earlier is that you can gradually expose yourself to higher and higher volumes of noise by simply increasing the volume of your masker.

Initially, set the volume at a low level. If you can tolerate this, increase it a little and get used to this by trying it on the same level either for an hour or in small bursts of a few minutes several times for part of a day. As you learn to tolerate one noise level, go on to a slightly higher volume and work your way up. This treatment can be very successful because the fear-arousing stimulus, the noise level, is entirely under your control.

If you want to try a masker, ask at your audiology clinic. If you have the opportunity to try a masker please try to persist with it for a while because, for most of our patients, relief from tinnitus does not come immediately.

4 Avoid difficult situations or leave when you can't cope

As discussed in Chapter 3, 'Overcoming anxiety', this is a very commonly used strategy. whilst it may have short term benefits (reduction of anxiety, avoidance of embarrassment, etc.), it will usually prove to bring about longer term costs. The most likely costs apart from disappointments and maybe feelings that you are letting yourself and other people down, are that such situations may become increasingly difficult to tolerate over time. In a sense you may learn to avoid more and more situations because you will have learned that you can't cope.

Another difficulty is that it may be very difficult to anticipate how you will be in any situation that induces feelings of apprehension. People with anxiety problems generally overestimate the anxiety they expect to suffer in situations in the future. Your experience will usually tell you that 'It wasn't as bad as I thought it would be'. By avoiding, you protect yourself from 'harm' but miss out on potential enjoyment. If this is a struggle for you, please try out the approaches described in Chapter 3

7 Imagery

Chapter goals

We hope that by the end of this chapter you will be able to understand more about the ways in which tinnitus causes you to become distressed. The noise is only the start, your reactions to it are more important. This is because although we can't take the noise away, we can show you how to reduce the problems which tinnitus causes.

The distress which tinnitus causes is, of course, not restricted to the immediate reactions which people have towards the noise. Many people complained that it wasn't the noise that was the problem, but the fact that they couldn't sleep, or were short tempered. These problems are dealt with elsewhere in the book.

This chapter will show how the 'image' which you have or the way that you 'label' the tinnitus affects the distress which it causes. In addition, we will suggest some ways of modifying the image so that it does not cause so much of a problem.

When we began to try to get to know our patients for the first time, we had firm ideas about the aspects of tinnitus which would be the most difficult for people to accept. It should come as no surprise to you to discover that many of our 'firm ideas' didn't last very long. If you share some of our misconceptions then the following section may help you to identify them for yourself.

If you agree with the following then write 'Agree' in the box at the end of each statement. However, if you do not then write 'Disagree'.

The answers are given at the end of the questionnaire.

1 We thought that the people with the loudest noise would be the most distressed

2 We thought that the type of noise would be particularly important.

3 Older people would always find tinnitus more difficult to live with than younger people.

4 People with tinnitus would be disturbed equally in all situations.

5 Tinnitus would always become less of a problem the longer it went on.

6 People who had someone that they could rely on for emotional support would always find tinnitus less of a problem.

7 The reaction of people to their tinnitus noise would be a good indication of the amount of disruption it would cause in their lives

The answers may surprise you because we found that it was only the Final statement (number 7) that helped us to help the majority of our patients. The other statements seem to be common sense; indeed, we had been told that they were important by the first tinnitus sufferers that we saw. These factors were important to some sufferers, but not to the majority of people with tinnitus.

Why was it that we began with a number of assumptions that we later dismissed? A partial answer is that most of the list came from the comments of the first patients that we saw, the majority of whom had been suffering great distress from their tinnitus for a long time. People who were able to adjust to the problem obviously didn't ask to be referred. When we began to speak to people who were living successfully with their problem, we saw that our patients had been telling us about their reaction to tinnitus, not the tinnitus itself. We began to look for other reasons for their distress. We eventually found that a major difference between the 'distressed' and 'non-distressed' patients was how they labelled their tinnitus.

This may seem to be a strange way to think about a problem which will obviously be unpleasant. However, remember that although some people said that one aspect of their tinnitus was causing their distress, other sufferers would give a different account. An example of this is the patient who said that it was the volume which was the problem; we found people who reported volume as great (or greater) who were able to live without great distress. We often found that the difference between them was that one group had been able to feel less 'threatened' by their tinnitus, they had given it an 'OK' label.

It may not seem to you that you have given your tinnitus a 'problem' label, not everyone does but we found that a great many of our patients had. The way that they sometimes came to recognise the label was to realise that although their tinnitus was with them much of the time they felt most distressed by it at particular times. When we asked them to close their eyes and think themselves back into the problem situation and tell us how they felt, they would often notice unpleasant emotions such as anger or fear. Patients would also tend to say that they had begun to perspire or had noticed that they were trembling. They said that they felt confused because they had been told that their problem wasn't life–threatening and they hadn't realised that it was making them frightened, anxious, angry etc. It was as though they understood the tinnitus with their head, but not their emotions.

The following list contains some of the bodily changes that people noticed when they began to think about their tinnitus:

1 tense muscles
2 their heart began to beat more quickly
3 they began to perspire
4 they began to feel warm
5 they began to blush
6 they felt dizzy or light–headed
7 they felt slight tingling in their fingers
8 a slight choking sensation
9 a slight headache
10 they had began to breathe more quickly
11 they were breathing more heavily

Obviously we don't expect that you will notice all (or even most) of these sensations. However, it may be helpful to take some time to notice how your body is feeling the next time that you are troubled by tinnitus.

In the chapter goals we said that the 'image' which you have of your tinnitus has an effect on how you feel. The sort of label which you give to your tinnitus is the result of the image that you have of it. This may seem complicated; it isn't, but it takes a little time to understand. This is because it's an unusual way to think about something that you think you know well.

It may be useful to review the ground that we have covered so far:

(a) When we concentrated on the tinnitus noise alone we didn't find that we could help individual patients because the problems which they said that tinnitus caused them varied so much.

(b) The more useful approach was to find out the reaction which people have towards their tinnitus because although many people said that their tinnitus was always present, they were not always distressed by it.

(c) The people who seek treatment tend to be distressed by their tinnitus. Therefore, we didn't find out that people could have the same sort of tinnitus as our patients but not be as distressed.

(d) The people who were not as distressed seemed to regard their tinnitus differently than the distressed people. This was reflected in the ways that they described their tinnitus to themselves. We called this the 'label' that they used.

(e) When people who were distressed by their tinnitus explained how they felt when their tinnitus was most troublesome, they sometimes noticed that they seemed to have become anxious or angry although they couldn't see a reason for doing so.

(f) A useful pointer for these emotions was to pay attention to any bodily changes, not on their thoughts or the tinnitus.

As we have said many times before it isn't the tinnitus that is often the main problem. The majority of the distress can come from your reactions to the tinnitus. The list of bodily changes reported by our patients show just how powerfully your emotions can affect you. However, our patients didn't want to be distressed and couldn't understand why; they seemed to have come to terms with their problems on one level, but not on another. They knew what the problem was and that it did not threaten their health, so why did they suddenly become upset?

The upset came on so suddenly that they hadn't noticed how it had begun. As we have said before they couldn't give a reason even when they had thought about it carefully. The problems seem to suddenly appear all at once, but often only at particular times. Indeed, one person said that it felt a little like the feeling they had when waking from a nightmare. This is a good way of showing how things that have been in the back of our mind can influence our emotions. Most people will admit to dreaming about things that have happened during the day or are similar to incidents that have occurred at some time in their lives. The content of their dreams is sometimes things that they would have liked to have done in real life but were not able to. However, some dreams contain unpleasant or upsetting images, the effect of which is to cause us to wake up suddenly and feel distressed.

When we asked people to try to notice the images that were going through their mind when they were most distressed, they sometimes noticed them for the first time. It came as quite a surprise to them that we didn't just mean words, but any image that came into their mind. The images were sometimes upsetting, but they seemed to be less threatening when they had been written down. Indeed, the patients sometimes couldn't believe that they had not realised how foolish the images were, until they had taken the time to work them through. The patient's emotions seemed to reflect the worst possible circumstances, not the person's actual situation.

We hope that the relationship between the tinnitus, the image and the subsequent emotion will seem clearer after you have read the following example:

Mrs L

When she attended her first appointment she said that she had not been able to go out and mix socially since her tinnitus began. This was because it was a constant loud rushing sound that upset her. If we could only take the noise away then she would be right again and not the prisoner that she felt herself to be. The link between the tinnitus noise and her emotions was explained to her.

During the appointment she agreed to recall a recent occasion that her tinnitus had caused her particular distress. When she had done so, she said that she felt hot and that her heart had begun to beat more quickly. She noticed that she was feeling anxious. The images that she noticed were of how her former friends would react to her. The tinnitus meant that she would find it more difficult to follow conversations, especially in social situations when several people were speaking at once.

Mrs L recognised that she had become distressed because she had reacted to the image of herself being seen as inadequate by her friends. The anxiety did not come from the image that 'I will find social situations more difficult than before' but from the image 'I will never be able to go out socially again because my friends won't want to be bothered with me'. This was the image that came into her mind each time that she thought about her social life or resuming her former friendships.

The image began to change as she began to challenge it in two ways: (**a**) when she became upset using a more realistic image instead of the one which cause her distress; (**b**) starting to meet her friends individually or in quieter surroundings than before.

Many of our patients find that when they begin to feel that they are able to control their tinnitus, it becomes much less of a problem. We have found that it is sometimes helpful to use mental images to help to get the feeling of starting to control your problem. This may seem to be strange at first, until you realise that we all use something similar at one time or another to help us solve all sorts of problems.

Think back to your childhood or listen to what young children say about their problems. Many children will admit to feeling frightened of quite ordinary things, not because of what it is but because of what they have told themselves about it. They soon begin to grow out of this and adults very rarely do it. However, when faced with unpleasant events, especially those which we find difficult to control, adults become anxious and the problem has a greater impact upon their lives than it rightly deserves to do.

The sounds of tinnitus are often similar to sounds in the world around us. Many sufferers when they have thought about it will agree that at least some of their sounds are something like sounds they have heard before. The major difference is, they say, that those sounds were 'out there' and could be 'tuned out'. Their tinnitus is produced 'in here' and so cannot be controlled. This means that they will always have the problem.

The research which has been done into tinnitus does not seem to show that the type of sound is important in predicting how much distress it will cause. Therefore, it may be that the attitude which the person holds towards the problem is an important influence in how much distress it will cause.

Write down a description of your tinnitus in as much detail as possible:

Now look at what you have just written and write down all of
the words which describe sounds (note if they are pleasant or
unpleasant, loud or soft, etc.)

| 1 | 2 | 3 |
| 4 | 5 | 6 |

Most people find it difficult to separate how they feel about the
sounds from what they are.

Let's take an example to make it clear what to do next.

Suppose that you have written:

1 *Bell* **2** *Hissing* **3** *Low hum*

Now think about the sound; in other circumstances could it be
less upsetting to you than it is at the moment?

Some of our patients readily agree that the sound of a bell can
be pleasant (a church bell for example) but not if it rings all the
time! Use the following checklist to help you to recognise and
challenge the 'problem' images.

Think about an occasion when your tinnitus has been particularly troublesome.

1 Try to think yourself **into the situation** rather than just
thinking about it. This means that you should try to concentrate
and get as complete a picture as you can. Include as many of the
following as you can:

   (**a**) any other sounds (conversations, music, traffic noise, etc.)
   (**b**) any tastes (were you having a meal or swimming?)
   (**c**) any sensations of touch (were you in a crowd?)
   (**d**) any perfumes or odours (were you in a garden?)
   (**e**) as many visual details as possible (not just 'flowers' but which
      variety, how tall, which colours, the shape of leaves and petals,
      etc.

2 Notice any bodily changes.

We find that it is often helpful for patients to keep a record of how
they feel each time they do this exercise. Therefore, put the date
at the top of the column and then put a tick by the feelings which
you noticed

	Date	Date	Date
1 Tense muscles			
2 Heart beating more quickly			
3 Increased perspiration			
4 Feeling warmer			
5 Blushing			
6 Dizzy or light–headed			
7 Slight tingling in your fingers			
8 Slight choking sensation			
9 Slight headache			
10 Breathing more quickly			
11 Breathing more heavily			
12 Feeling slightly upset			
13 Feeling frightened			
14 Feeling 'on edge'			
15 Feeling relaxed			
16 Feeling happy			
17 Feeling better than before			

If you noticed emotional or bodily changes, try to remember the images which went through your mind immediately before the changes. Write down the content of the image:

Date _____

Date _____

Date _____

When the images came into you mind did you notice that your emotions began to change at the same time?

Challenge the statements that you have just written down.

Is the image true?

Is the image reasonable?

If it was about someone else would you still accept it?

Is the image always true for everyone?

Write down the 'OK' images and use them to challenge the 'problem' images each time that they occur. Remember that the images have to be challenged not only by what you think, but also by testing out your '**OK**' images in the real world. Mrs L. thought that she was able to resume her friendships but could only prove this to herself by taking sensible steps towards her goal.

A helpful technique (to supplement the 'real life' practice) is to use the relaxation exercises (given at the end of the book) to let your mind relax. Allow a pleasant image to come into your mind and practise this until you can bring it into your mind quickly. Then think yourself into a problem situation **as soon as** the upsetting images come into your mind, challenge it by switching your mind onto the pleasant image.

This is often a time-consuming exercise, but many people find that the effort is worth it. They are able to bring the pleasant image into their mind in any situation, not just when they are relaxing. We hope that you will be able to use images to reduce the distress which tinnitus causes. However, remember it may take a lot of practice, so please don't feel discouraged if you don't get it right the first time.

8 Relaxation assessment

To find out how well you are able to use the relaxation exercises rate how relaxed you feel **in general** each day. To do this rate the **relaxation** from 0–100%.

Therefore, if you are not at all relaxed for any part of the day you would score 0% However, if you are totally relaxed all the time then you would score 100%

Try to rate yourself about the same time each day for the next three weeks on the table below:

DAY	SCORE	DAY	SCORE
1		11	
2		12	
3		13	
4		14	
5		15	
6		16	
7		17	
8		18	
9		19	
10		20	
21			

As you become more skilled at using the relaxation exercises, try rating how tense you were:
   (**a**) Before (or during) a difficult situation
   (**b**) Following your use of the relaxation exercises

Remember: If your tinnitus causes most distress when you are sitting quietly (with little on your mind), then you may find some of the other approaches more useful. However, when you feel more confident about sitting and listening to the noise, come back to this section.

Relaxation instructions

So that the relaxation exercises are of most help please make sure that you have thought about the 'obvious' problems, which are often overlooked.

The room Have you chosen the room in which you are going to relax with care:
- Is it quiet?
- Are you going to be disturbed?
- Do you feel 'comfortable' in the room, has it got the right atmosphere?
- Is it uncomfortably hot or cold?
- Can you lie down easily when doing the exercises?

The person.
- Don't try to do the exercises if you are hungry or have just eaten.
- Don't worry about your performance or whether you are 'doing the relaxation properly'.
- Don't see the exercises as something which will be a struggle. Just give yourself time to learn ...
- Try to breathe through your nose and use your stomach muscles as you inhale and exhale.
- Try to breath slowly and regularly ... Don't take lots of quick deep breaths as you may start to feel sick or dizzy and so make yourself even more tense.

The exercises

We hope that by doing the exercises you will begin to notice the difference betueen tense and relaxed muscles. When people have mastered this skill they are often surprised at how often each day they tense their muscles.

- Make yourself as comfortable as you can.
- Lie flat on a bed or the floor and put a pillow under your head, or settle into a comfortable chair.
- Take off your shoes (and spectacles if you wear them).
- Loosen any tight clothing.
- Relax your arms by your side and have your legs uncrossed.
- Close your eyes.
- Take a moment to notice how you feel before starting to relax.

The programme of relaxation always follows the same course,

starting with your feet and working up through your body. This is so that the exercises are easy to remember. We hope that you will be able to use the relaxation at will and so feel more confident, independent, and in control of your problem.

– Begin to breathe in and out **slowly and easily without effort**
– **Remember, you cannot force yourself to relax ... you just make yourself more and more tense.**
– Keep breathing rhythmically, and perhaps notice the tense feelings starting to reduce.
– Let your body begin to relax.
– When you have started to feel a little calmer begin to let your mind focus on your body and how it feels ... not the tinnitus!
– Begin to think about your feet and ankles.
– **Remember, relaxation is a skill which involves your mind and body ... many people find that as they become more skilled they can concentrate upon the pleasant sensations of relaxation and so exclude the tinnitus.**
– Begin to tense the muscles in your feet and ankles by curling your toes towards your head.
– Gently and progressively feel your muscles begin to stretch and the tension slowly increase in your feet and ankles.
– Hold this feeling for a count of two ...
– Let the tension go completely.
– Notice how limp and relaxed your feet seem to be.
– Take a few seconds to notice the difference between the feelings of tension and relaxation in your muscles.
– Allow your feet to continue to relax ... they may begin to seem heavier and roll outwards ... this is normal and natural, so just allow it to happen.
– If you wish to do so tense and relax your feet again as we just did ... make sure that you take time to notice the difference between unpleasant tension and the soothing sensation of relaxation.
– Now let your mind concentrate on the muscles of your calves.
– As we did before, slowly and gently tense the muscles in your lower legs ... begin to raise both legs up in front of you.
– Hold this feeling for a count of two ...
– Let the tension go completely.
– Notice how limp and relaxed your calf muscles seem to be.
– Take a few seconds to notice the difference between the feelings of tension and relaxation.
– Feel the tension begin to drain away from your calves and your feet. As before, relaxed muscles often feel heavier than when they are tense ... so if you notice this don't be anxious, it is normal and natural.

- If you wish to do so tense and relax your calves again as we just did ... make sure that you take time to notice the difference between unpleasant tension and the soothing sensation of relaxation.
- Let your mind move up your body and begin to notice the tension in your thigh muscles.
- Start to make the muscles tense by progressively pushing the tops of your legs together until you can notice the difference.
- Hold this feeling for a count of two ...
- Let the tension go completely.
- Notice how limp and relaxed your thighs seem to be.
- Take a few seconds to notice the difference between the feelings of tension and relaxation in your muscles as we just did ... make sure that you take time to notice the difference between unpleasant tension and the soothing sensation of relaxation.
- Let your mind move up your body and begin to notice the tension in your thigh muscles.
- Start to make the muscles tense by progressively pushing the tops of your legs together until you can notice the difference.
- Hold this feeling for a count of two ...
- Let the tension go completely.
- Notice how limp and relaxed your thighs seem to be.
- Take a few seconds to notice the difference between the feelings of tension and relaxation in your muscles.
- If you wish to do so tense and relax your thighs again as we just did ... make sure that you take time to notice the difference between unpleasant tension and the soothing sensation of relaxation.
- Next begin to tense the muscles of your hips and lower back.
- You can do this by slowly and gently squeezing your buttocks together.
- Hold this feeling for a count of two...
- Let the tension go completely.
- Notice how limp and relaxed your back and hips seem to be.
- Take a few seconds to notice the difference between the feelings of tension and relaxation in your muscles.
- If you wish to do so tense and relax your back and hips again as we just did ... make sure that you take time to notice the difference between unpleasant tension and the soothing sensation of relaxation.
- The exercises now move up to the muscles of your stomach and chest.
- Take a few seconds to focus your mind onto this area of your body ... now that you are becoming more familiar with the sensation of tension, can you notice that the muscles are less relaxed than you thought when you started the exercises?
- Progressively tense the muscles in your chest and stomach ... imagine that you are about to receive a blow in your stomach; take in a breath and at the same time, pull in your stomach.

- Notice how unpleasant the feeling of tension is.
- Hold this feeling for a count of two ...
- Breath out and let the tension go completely.
- Notice how limp and relaxed you are starting to become.
- Take a few seconds to notice the difference between the feelings of tension and relaxation in your muscles.
- Notice the tension leaving your chest and stomach ... feel the sensations of tightness leave your body.
- Allow your breathing to become effortless and even ... rhythmic and relaxed.
- If you wish to do so tense and relax again ... make sure that you take time to notice the difference between unpleasant tension and the soothing sensation of relaxation ... Between stressed forced breathing and when it is effortless, rhythmic and relaxed.
- You can now move up to your hands and arms ... Notice any tension ... focus your mind and concentrate on the muscles.
- Slowly make your hands into tight fists.
- Then hold your arms straight out in front of you with your hands still in tight fists.
- Hold this feeling for a count of two ...
- Let the tension go completely and allow your arms and hands to rest lightly by your side.
- Notice how limp and relaxed your arms and hands have become.
- Take a few seconds to notice the difference between the feelings of tension and relaxation.
- If you wish to do so tense and relax your arms and hands as we just did... make sure that you take time to notice the difference between unpleasant tension and the soothing sensation of relaxation.
- As before, relaxed muscles often feel heavier than when they are tense ... so if you notice this don't be anxious, it is normal and natural.
- Neck and shoulder muscles are often the most easily noticed as being tense and painful, therefore, it should be easier to notice the difference when they are relaxed.
- Draw your shoulders in towards your ears and then pull your shoulder blades towards your spine.
- Hold this feeling for a count of two ...
- Tense your neck muscles even more by slightly tipping your head back.
- Hold the tension for a count of two...
- Let the tension go completely.
- Notice how relaxed your neck and shoulders have become.
- Take a few seconds to notice the difference between the feelings of tension and relaxation in your muscles.
- If you wish tense and relax again ... make sure that you take time to notice the difference between unpleasant tension and the soothing

sensation of relaxation.
- Feel all of your muscles relaxing more and more deeply.
- The final group of muscles are those of the face.
- Notice any tension, however slight ... direct your thought to your face ... try to become aware of little else than the sensation of discomfort which tense muscles cause.
- Frown as hard as you can.
- Hold this feeling and tense the muscles in your jaw by biting hard.
- Feel the unpleasant sensations as they begin to increase.
- Hold this feeling for a count of two ...
- Let the tension go completely and let your jaw drop.
- Notice how limp and relaxed you have become compared to how you felt when you began the exercises.
- Take a few seconds to notice the difference between the feelings of tension and relaxation in your muscles.
- If you wish to do so tense and relax your muscles again as we just did ... make sure that you take time to notice the difference between unpleasant tension and the soothing sensation of relaxation.
- The final stage is to let your mind take stock of your whole body ... Notice that your muscles may feel heavy and perhaps for the first time you may feel how the chair or bed or floor has begun to support your body rather than the tension in your muscles.
- You may feel as though you are floating; don't worry, this sometimes happens and is a natural part of becoming relaxed.
- Let your mind drift onto pleasant images; relax and put the worries of life to one side; just enjoy the pleasant feelings of relaxation.
- Take some time to slowly leave the pleasant feelings of relaxation and become more aware of your surroundings ... until you are fully alert.
- **Make sure that you don't stand up too quickly as you may feel a bit light-headed.**

Quick relaxation

One of the most important things to remember about relaxation is that it is a skill that, when learned can help you in a variety of troublesome situations. The problem is that the long version, although effective, takes some time, and is difficult to use in social situations. The following relaxation exercises are easier to learn and use. However, we recommend that you begin to learn the short cut to relaxation after you have learned the full version.

The major difference between this and the other version is that you don't need to tense your muscles.

- Begin by sitting well back in a comfortable chair, with your thighs and back supported.
- As we said before, it is just about impossible to 'force' yourself to relax. Therefore, start your sessions by slowly breathing out. Allow your body to get the message that it is all right if the muscles become less tense.
- Begin by taking slow, unforced breaths, using a regular rhythm.
- After you have settled into an easy and pleasant routine allow yourself to relax a little bit more each time you breathe out.
- Feel the tension in your muscles begin to ease away.
- Notice that as your body becomes less tense your mind seems to relax, problems become less urgent and upsetting.
- As you begin to reduce your tension, you may notice some of the same things happening as when you did the longer exercises. You know that feeling a bit heavier, or feeling yourself being supported by the chair, or feeling a bit warmer, etc. are normal and natural and nothing to worry about.
- The golden rule is to take things at your own pace; the prize is that you are able to help yourself feel better, not that you can do the exercises for longer, or more quickly than anyone else.
- Keep breathing regularly and easily try saying 'relax' to yourself as you notice the tension continue to leave your body.
- As we did before, start to deepen the relaxation by concentrating on individual parts of your body.
- Think of your feet, allow the tension to flow away. As your feet relax they may roll outwards; this is expected, so you don't need to get anxious about it.
- Take a few moments, and notice how much more you could relax when you allow your body to do so.
- Move your attention to your calves; imagine the muscles becoming floppy and relaxed.
- Take the time that you need for your calves to fully relax.
- Keep breathing regularly and easily; try saying 'relax' to yourself as you notice the tension continue to leave your body.
- When you feel ready, begin to notice the tension in your thigh muscles; allow your legs to fall apart.
- As you continue to breathe easily and regularly, imagine the tension draining away from your thighs, your calves and your feet.
- The next areas of relaxation are the muscles of your hips and lower back. Think of the tension slowly fading away and being replaced by the warm and pleasant sensations of relaxation.
- When it's comfortable to do so, think of the unpleasant sensation of tension in the muscles of your stomach and chest.
- Allow any tightness to leave your chest.
- Keep breathing regularly and easily; try saying 'relax' to yourself as

you notice the tension continue to leave your body.

- Think about your arms and hands, are they even slightly tense?
- Allow them to rest comfortably on your lap or the arms of the chair.
- They may feel heavy as they relax; this is natural so don't worry about it, just notice how pleasant the feeling of relaxation is.
- When you are ready, think about the tension in your shoulders and neck. Allow your head to drop forward, and let your shoulders ease downwards.
- Notice the tension begin to flow away; feel the muscles relaxing more and more deeply.
- Keep breathing regularly and easily try saying 'relax' to yourself as you notice the tension continue to leave your body.
- The final area of relaxation is the same as with the other exercises. Think about the muscles in your face, and try to pinpoint any tension.
- Relax your forehead and let your jaw drop. Notice the tension disappearing as you breathe slowly and easily with a natural rhythm.
- When you have been able to relax, let any tension from your body ease away. The sensations of relaxation are often very pleasant, so let yourself relax and let your mind drift.
- Notice how limp and relaxed you have become, compared to how you felt when you began the exercises.
- Take a few seconds to notice the difference between the feelings of tension and relaxation in your muscles. Notice that your muscles may feel heavy and perhaps for the first time you may feel how the chair has begun to support your body rather than the tension in your muscles.
- You may feel as though you are floating;don't worry, this sometimes happens and is natural a part of becoming relaxed.
- Let your mind drift on to pleasant images; relax and put the worries of life to one side just enjoy the pleasant feelings of relaxation.
- Take some time to slowly leave the pleasant feelings of relaxation and become more aware of your surroundings until you are fully alert.
- **Make sure that you don't stand up too quickly as you may feel a bit light-headed.**
- **Taking things a bit more slowly may be useful at other times as well ... it may prevent you from becoming tense in the first place!**

9 Your ear

To help you to understand and cope with your tinnitus we have
included a short section which explains how your ear is made and
how sound is turned into hearing. However, you don't have to
'plough through' this if you find it boring (or confusing). Indeed,
some of our patients say that they are happier not knowing a lot
about their ear. They prefer to concentrate on finding ways of
overcoming the problems which tinnitus causes in their lives.

A good way of starting to understand how your ear works is to
follow the same route as the sound, that is, to start on the outside
and move in towards the brain.

The ear is divided into three sections: (**a**) the external ear; (**b**)
the middle ear; (**c**) the inner ear. It is also important to remember
that the ear is responsible for giving information about balance
as well as allowing you to hear.

The external ear

The major parts of the ear which you can see are called the **pinna**
and the **external auditory meatus** (ear canal).

The middle ear

This is separated from the external ear by the ear drum (**tympanic membrane**) and it contains the three small bones (**auditory ossicles**): the hammer (**malleus**), anvil (**incus**) and stir-
rup (**stapes**). In addition, the nerve of taste (**chorda tympani**)
can be found in this area.

The inner ear

The **cochlea** is filled with fluid and contains cells which are
sensitive to changes in the pressure of the fluid. The inner ear

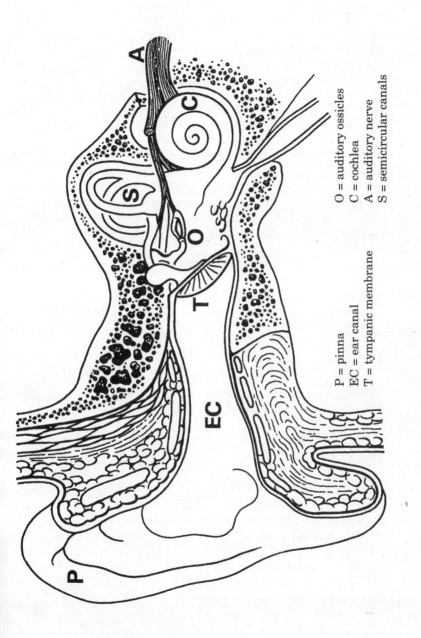

P = pinna
EC = ear canal
T = tympanic membrane

O = auditory ossicles
C = cochlea
A = auditory nerve
S = semicircular canals

also contains the semicircular canals which are responsible for your sense of balance.

Sound is funnelled by the **pinna** (**P**) through the **ear canal** (**EC**) to the **tympanic membrane** (**T**) which vibrates with the sound. The **auditory ossicles** (**O**) move because of this vibration. The **stapes** presses against the **cochlea** (**C**).Cells in the **cochlea** which connect with the **auditory nerve** (**A**) convert the vibrations into nerve impulses. The **semicircular canals** (**S**) give you your sense of balance.

Glossary

We know that many people find that going to hospital, even for tests, is a bit frightening and confusing. This means that they often don't ask the staff to explain words that they have used. The following list contains some that may have been used when you were at the hospital. We hope that it will help you not to worry. The problem with lists like this is that the word that you thought you would look up when you came home is always missing! Therefore, if you feel confused or you don't quite understand what is going on, ask the staff to explain. They won't think that you are wasting their time because if you don't understand what they are asking you to do, your treatment may be more of a problem to them later on.

The names of the parts of the ear are not all given in the glossary, but can be found in the section called 'Your ear'.

ACOUSTIC NERVE: this is the nerve which connects the ear and brain. As your ear only detects sounds, your brain has to make sense of them in order that you can make sense of what you hear.

ACOUSTIC TRAUMA: this seems to be one of the most important single causes of tinnitus; the inside of the ear is damaged because of a very loud noise. You can think of it as being 'overloaded' by the sound.

ANXIETY: this is a common feeling, especially when we are faced with a problem of some sort. The feeling of anxiety can become a problem if we begin to have our lives restricted because of fears which become out of proportion to the original problem. Psychological treatments often help to overcome anxiety or reduce the problems to a minimum (see chapter 3).

AUDIOGRAM: This is the chart which shows the range of sounds which you could hear when you were tested (see Audiometry).

AURICLE: this is the part of the ear that you can see and recognise as an ear.

AUDIOMETRY: when people attend clinics for treatment of hearing problems they are often given a hearing test. The name given to the process for scientifically investigating how well you are able to hear is Audoimetry.

AUDITORY CANAL: this is the tube which connects your ear drum to the part of the ear that you can see (auricle).

BEHAVIOUR THERAPY: this is the name given to a psychological treatment for 'emotional' and other problems. It differs from some other methods because it regards problems as being produced by the person learning an inappropriate way of dealing with their problems. Therefore, it does not look for 'unconscious' drives or impulses to explain why a person has difficulties in their life.

BINAURAL: this is a short way of saying 'both ears'.

COCHLEA: this is found in the inner ear. It is a tube filled with liquid and is particularly important, as it contains the part of your ear responsible for turning sound vibrations into nerve impulses. In addition, it is connected to the vestibular system.

COCHLEA IMPLANT: when a person has become totally deaf after having good hearing, they can sometimes benefit from a particular operation. The surgeon fits a small electrical device which although it does not restore their hearing, can help them to better understand conversations and other sounds.

COGNITIVE THERAPY: this is a similar approach to psychological problems as behaviour therapy (see above). The main difference between them is that cognitive therapy concentrates on how you are thinking about the problems and tries to help you think them through clearly.

COMBINATION INSTRUMENT: as with a hearing aid, this device is worn in or behind your ear. However, it has a tinnitus masker and a hearing aid.

CONDUCTIVE DEAFNESS: this is produced by damage or disease of the middle ear. This prevents the sound from reaching the inner ear.

DECIBEL (dB): the precise definition of this often heard term is complicated and confusing. Therefore, it may be more helpful to remember that: (a) the smallest noticeable change in sound intensity is about 3 decibels (b) a change of 10 decibel usually seems to be a doubling of loudness.

DEPRESSION: this can be a feeling of being 'down in the dumps' or a more serious problem. The depressed person can often get over the problem themselves or with some help from their friends or family. However, if the problem doesn't seem to be getting better then it is important to see your doctor who may treat you themselves, or may refer you for more specialist help (see chapter 4).

EAR CANAL: see 'Your ear'

EAR DRUM (TYMPANIC MEMBRANE): see 'Your ear'

EAR MOULD: this is a piece of plastic which fits into your ear and onto a hearing aid (or tinnitus masker or combination instrument) to allow the sound to be heard more clearly.

ELECTRICAL SUPPRESSION: this is a way of trying to reduce the tinnitus by using electricity.

HERTZ (Hz): this is a term which shows how many cycles per second have occurred. You will often find this used in connection with electrical equipment. As an example, the frequency of some radio stations is shown on the set in kHz or MHz meaning the number of hundreds or thousands of times per second that the radio waves have completed a cycle (from high to low then high, etc.).

HYPERACUSIS: you may hear this used by your doctor. This isn't some thing that you need to worry about, it simply means that noise levels which would not cause distress to the majority of people are troublesome or cause discomfort.

INNER EAR (LABYRINTH): see 'Your ear'

MASKER: this is a small device that looks very much like a hearing aid. However, instead of making it easier to hear, the masker makes a noise which can 'drown out' the tinnitus. Some sufferers find that a masker (or using a personal stereo with the volume high) can be a great help. We find that they tend to be used at night to help sufferers to get to sleep.

MENIERE'S DISEASE: this is an unpleasant condition which causes the sufferer to have attacks of vertigo. In addition, short episodes of hearing loss or tinnitus occur.The precise cause is not well understood, but it is known to be a result of disturbance to the inner ear (see 'Your ear').

MIDDLE EAR: see 'Your ear'

MONAURAL: this means 'one ear'.

NOISE–INDUCED TINNITUS: This is a common cause of tinnitus as its name suggests, meaning tinnitus produced by a loud noise.

OSSICLES: see 'Your ear'

OTOTOXIC SUBSTANCE: this is any chemical that can cause your hearing to become impaired.

PRESBYACUSIS: this is the name for the loss of hearing which is the result of age.

PULSATILE TINNITUS: as it's name suggests, this form of tinnitus has a regular form. This sometimes seems to be related to the pulses in the blood vessels near to the ear.

RESIDUAL INHIBITION: if a burst of sound is delivered into the ear, then the tinnitus sound may be reduced or in some cases stopped.

SEMI–CIRCULAR CANALS: see 'Your ear'

SENSORY–NEURAL DEAFNESS: this is the name for deafness which is the result of damage to the cochlea (see 'Your ear')

SENSORY–NEURAL TINNITUS: this is the name given to tinnitus caused by problems occurring in the inner ear (see above).

SIBILANTS: these are the hissing sounds of spoken words; they are only found in consonants. If you cannot hear them you will find conversations more difficult.

SYRINGING: this is a means of removing excessive ear wax by syringing water into the affected part of your ear.

TINNITUS MASKER: this is a small battery–driven device which looks like a hearing aid. The tinnitus masker is worn in or behind your ear and is intended to make enough acceptable noise to overcome the sound of your tinnitus.

TYMPANIC MEMBRANE: see 'Your ear'

VESTIBULAR APPARATUS: this is the part of your ear which helps you to know that you are balanced and stable.

VERTIGO: this is a feeling of dizziness often accompanied by feeling sick. The people who have this problem often complain that they or the world around them is spinning.

Recommended reading

Blackburn, I. (1987) *Coping with depression*. Chambers, Edinburgh.
Burns, D. (1981) *Feeling good: the new mood therapy*. Signet, New York.
Hambly, K. (1983) *Overcoming tension*. Sheldon Press, London.

Although not written for tinnitus sufferers, all of the books are intended to help people to overcome the sort of distress which tinnitus causes.

Useful addresses

BRITISH TINNITUS ASSOCIATION
c/o Royal National Institute for the Deaf, 105 Gower Street, London
WC1E 6AH **also** 14–18 West Bar Green, Sheffield S1 2DA

THE OPEN DOOR ASSOCIATION
447 Pensby Road, Heswall, Wirral, Merseyside LR1 9PQ

This is an association which provides information to people who have
anxiety problems, particularly people who find that anxiety makes it
hard for them to go out.

RNID TINNITUS SUPPORT SERVICE
Royal National Institute for the Deaf, 105 Gower Street, London
WC1E 6AH Tel: 071 387 8033

RNID TINNITUS HELPLINE
0345 090210 (Voice & Text)